Allergy and Asthma in Otolaryngology

Editors

DANIEL M. BESWICK
SARAH K. WISE

OTOLARYNGOLOGIC CLINICS OF NORTH AMERICA

www.oto.theclinics.com

Consulting Editor
SUJANA S. CHANDRASEKHAR

April 2024 • Volume 57 • Number 2

ELSEVIER

1600 John F. Kennedy Boulevard • Suite 1800 • Philadelphia, Pennsylvania, 19103-2899

http://www.oto.theclinics.com

OTOLARYNGOLOGIC CLINICS OF NORTH AMERICA Volume 57, Number 2
April 2024 ISSN 0030-6665, ISBN-13: 978-0-443-12963-6

Editor: Stacy Eastman
Developmental Editor: Malvika Shah

Otolaryngologic Clinics of North America (ISSN 0030-6665) is published bimonthly by Elsevier, Inc., 360 Park Avenue South, New York, NY 10010-1710. Months of issue are February, April, June, August, October, and December. Business and Editorial Offices: 1600 John F. Kennedy Blvd., Suite 1800, Philadelphia, PA 19103-2899. Customer Service Office: 6277 Sea Harbor Drive, Orlando, FL 32887-4800. Periodicals postage paid at New York, NY and additional mailing offices. Subscription prices are $478.00 per year (US individuals), $100.00 per year (US & Canadian student/resident), $623.00 per year (Canadian individuals), $679.00 per year (international individuals), $270.00 per year (international student/resident). For institutional access pricing please contact Customer Service via the contact information below. Foreign air speed delivery is included in all *Clinics*' subscription prices. All prices are subject to change without notice. **POSTMASTER:** Send address changes to *Otolaryngologic Clinics of North America*, Elsevier Health Sciences Division, Subscription Customer Service, 3251 Riverport Lane, Maryland Heights, MO 63043. **Telephone: 1-800-654-2452 (U.S. and Canada); 314-447-8871 (outside U.S. and Canada). Fax: 314-447-8029. E-mail: journalscustomerservice-usa@elsevier.com (for print support); journalsonlinesupport-usa@elsevier.com (for online support).**

Reprints. For copies of 100 or more of articles in this publication, please contact the Commercial Reprints Department, Elsevier Inc., 360 Park Avenue South, New York, NY 10010-1710. Tel.: 212-633-3874; Fax: 212-633-3820; E-mail: reprints@elsevier.com.

Otolaryngologic Clinics of North America is also published in Spanish by McGraw-Hill Interamericana Editores S.A., P.O. Box 5-237, 06500 Mexico D.F., Mexico.

Otolaryngologic Clinics of North America is covered in *MEDLINE/PubMed (Index Medicus), Current Contents/Clinical Medicine, Excerpta Medica, BIOSIS, Science Citation Index,* and *ISI/BIOMED.*

Contributors

CONSULTING EDITOR

SUJANA S. CHANDRASEKHAR, MD, FAAO-HNS, FAOS, FACS
Consulting Editor, *Otolaryngologic Clinics of North America*, President, American
Otological Society, Past President, American Academy of Otolaryngology-Head and Neck
Surgery, Partner, ENT & Allergy Associates, LLP, Clinical Professor, Department of
Otolaryngology-Head and Neck Surgery, Zucker School of Medicine at Hofstra-Northwell,
Clinical Associate Professor, Department of Otolaryngology-Head and Neck Surgery,
Icahn School of Medicine at Mount Sinai, New York, New York

EDITORS

DANIEL M. BESWICK, MD
Associate Professor, Department of Otolaryngology–Head and Neck Surgery, University
of California, Los Angeles, Los Angeles, California

SARAH K. WISE, MD, MSCR
Professor, Department of Otolaryngology–Head and Neck Surgery, Emory University
Hospital Midtown, Emory University, Atlanta, Georgia

AUTHORS

OMAR G. AHMED, MD
Assistant Clinical Member, Academic Institute; Assistant Professor of Otolaryngology,
Research Institute, Otolaryngology–Head and Neck Surgery, Houston Methodist Hospital,
Houston, Texas

ABDULRAHMAN ALENEZI, MD, FRCSC
Instructor of Otolaryngology, Department of Otolaryngology–Head and Neck Surgery,
Johns Hopkins School of Medicine, Johns Hopkins Outpatient Center, Baltimore,
Maryland

DHANYA ASOKUMAR, BS
Medical Student, Department of Otolaryngology–Head and Neck Surgery, University of
Michigan, Ann Arbor, Michigan

THOMAS F. BARRETT, MD
Division of Rhinology and Anterior Skull Base Surgery, Department of Otolaryngology–
Head and Neck Surgery, Washington University School of Medicine, St Louis, Missouri

MICHAEL S. BENNINGER, MD
Professor and Chair, Department of Otolaryngology–Head and Neck Surgery, Cleveland
Clinic Lerner College of Medicine, Head and Neck Institute, The Cleveland Clinic,
Cleveland, Ohio

DANIEL M. BESWICK, MD
Associate Professor, Department of Otolaryngology–Head and Neck Surgery, University of California, Los Angeles, Los Angeles, California

KODY G. BOLK, MD
Senior Associate, Department of Otolaryngology–Head and Neck Surgery, Emory University Hospital Midtown, Atlanta, Georgia

SUKHMANI BOPARAI, MBBS, MD
Fellow, UAB Division of Pulmonary, Allergy, and Critical Care Medicine, University of Alabama at Birmingham, Pulmonary and Critical Care Medicine, Birmingham, Alabama

BRIAN H. CAMERON, MD
Resident, Department of Otorhinolaryngology–Head and Neck Surgery, McGovern Medical School, The University of Texas Health Science Center, Houston, Texas

DINESH CHHETRI, MD
Vice-Chair of the UCLA Department of Head and Neck Surgery, Director of the UCLA Swallowing Disorders Program and the UCLA Head and Neck Cancer Survivorship Program, Co-director of the UCLA Voice Center, Laryngology Program, University of California Los Angeles, Los Angeles, California

JOHN D. CLINGER, MD
Associate Professor, Department of Otolaryngology, Wake Forest School of Medicine, Winston-Salem, North Carolina

DAVID B. CORRY, MD
Professor, Department of Medicine, Biology of Inflammation Center, Baylor College of Medicine, Houston, Texas

CECELIA DAMASK, DO
Associate Clinical Professor, Department of Otolaryngology, Orlando ENT & Allergy, University of Central Florida, Orlando, Florida

JOHN M. DELGAUDIO, MD
Professor, Department of Otolaryngology–Head and Neck Surgery, Emory University Hospital Midtown, Atlanta, Georgia

ROHIT D. DIVEKAR, MBBS, PhD
Assistant Professor, Division of Allergic Diseases, Department of Medicine, Mayo Clinic, Rochester, Minnesota

THOMAS S. EDWARDS, MD
Assistant Professor, Department of Otolaryngology–Head and Neck Surgery, Emory University Hospital Midtown, Atlanta, Georgia

GARY A. FALCETANO, PA-C
Scientific Affairs Manager – Allergy, Immuno Diagnostics Division, Thermo Fisher Scientific, Portage, Michigan

CHRISTINE FRANZESE, MD
Professor, Director of Allergy, Department of Otolaryngology–Head and Neck Surgery, University of Missouri-Columbia, Columbia, Missouri

AMARBIR S. GILL, MD
Assistant Professor, Department of Otolaryngology–Head and Neck Surgery, University of Michigan, Ann Arbor, Michigan

SHAINA W. GONG, MD
Resident, Department of Otorhinolaryngology–Head and Neck Surgery, McGovern Medical School, The University of Texas Health Science Center, Houston, Texas

PAAVALI HANNIKAINEN, BS
Medical Student, Sidney Kimmel Medical College, Thomas Jefferson University, Philadelphia, Pennsylvania

ELINA JERSCHOW, MD, MSc
Professor of Immunology and Medicine, Chair, Division of Allergic Diseases, Department of Medicine, Mayo Clinic, Rochester, Minnesota

CHASE KAHN, MD
Physician Resident, Professor and Vice Chair, Department of Otolaryngology, Thomas Jefferson University, Philadelphia, Pennsylvania

JEAN KIM, MD, PhD
Associate Professor, Department of Otolaryngology–Head and Neck Surgery, Associate Professor, Department of Medicine, Allergy and Clinical Immunology, The Johns Hopkins University School of Medicine, Baltimore, Maryland

AMBER U. LUONG, MD, PhD
Professor, Department of Otorhinolaryngology–Head and Neck Surgery, Vice Chair for Academic Affairs, Center for Immunology and Autoimmune Diseases, Institute of Molecular Medicine, McGovern Medical School, The University of Texas Health Science Center, Houston, Texas

HANNA K. MANDL, BS
Medical Student, University of California, Los Angeles, David Geffen School of Medicine, Los Angeles, California

JOSE L. MATTOS, MD, MPH
Associate Professor, Department of Otolaryngology–Head and Neck Surgery, University of Virginia, Charlottesville, Virginia

JESSA E. MILLER, MD
Physician, Department of Otolaryngology–Head and Neck Surgery, University of California, Los Angeles, Los Angeles, California

JAMES W. MIMS, MD
Professor, Department of Otolaryngology, Wake Forest School of Medicine, Winston-Salem, North Carolina

NAINIKA NANDA, MD
HS Clinical Instructor, Department of Head and Neck Surgery, University of California Los Angeles, Los Angeles, California

ERIN K. O'BRIEN, MD
Associate Professor, Department of Otolaryngology–Head and Neck Surgery, Mayo Clinic, Rochester, Minnesota

JESSICA M.L. PAGEL, AB
Medical Student, University of Virginia School of Medicine, Charlottesville, Virginia

KUNJAN B. PATEL, MD
Resident, Department of Otolaryngology, Wake Forest School of Medicine, Winston-Salem, North Carolina

HANNAN QURESHI, MD
Professor, Vice Chair, Clinical Fellow and Instructor, Department of Otolaryngology–Head and Neck Surgery, Johns Hopkins School of Medicine, Johns Hopkins Outpatient Center, Baltimore, Maryland

MURUGAPPAN RAMANATHAN Jr, MD
Professor, Vice Chair, Department of Otolaryngology–Head and Neck Surgery, Johns Hopkins School of Medicine, Johns Hopkins Outpatient Baltimore, Maryland, USA

LAUREN T. ROLAND, MD, MSCI
Assistant Professor, Division of Rhinology and Anterior Skull Base Surgery, Department of Otolaryngology–Head and Neck Surgery, Washington University School of Medicine, St Louis, Missouri

GEORGE M. SOLOMON, MD
Associate Professor of Medicine, UAB Division of Pulmonary, Allergy, and Critical Care Medicine, University of Alabama at Birmingham, Pulmonary and Critical Care Medicine, Director, UAB Adult PCD and Bronchiectasis Programs, Director, Associate Director, UAB Pulmonary and Critical Care Fellowship, UAB CF Therapeutics Development Network Center, Associate Scientist, Gregory Fleming James CF Research Center, Birmingham, Alabama

ELINA TOSKALA, MD, PhD, MBA
Physician Resident, Department of Otolaryngology, Thomas Jefferson University, Philadelphia, Pennsylvania

DARRYN WAUGH, PhD
Professor, Department of Earth and Planetary Sciences, Kennedy Krieger School of Arts and Sciences, Johns Hopkins University, Baltimore, Maryland

SARAH K. WISE, MD, MSCR
Professor, Department of Otolaryngology–Head and Neck Surgery, Emory University Hospital Midtown, Emory University, Atlanta, Georgia

BENJAMIN ZAITCHIK, PhD
Professor, Department of Earth and Planetary Sciences, Kennedy Krieger School of Arts and Sciences, Johns Hopkins University, Baltimore, Maryland

Contents

Foreword: Runny Noses, Postnasal Drip, and Wheezing   xiii

Sujana S. Chandrasekhar

Preface: Allergy and Asthma in Otolaryngology: Current Management Paradigms   xv

Daniel M. Beswick and Sarah K. Wise

Allergic Rhinitis, Rhinosinusitis, and Asthma: Connections Across the Unified Airway   171

Paavali Hannikainen, Chase Kahn, and Elina Toskala

> The upper and lower airways are referred to as a single, integrated entity in the unified airway paradigm. When an allergen exposure occurs, the body responds locally and systemically, causing inflammation in other respiratory sites. As a result, asthmatic lower airway inflammation frequently coexists with upper airway inflammation, such as allergic rhinitis. Otolaryngologists are in a unique position to detect undiagnosed lower airway illness, start the proper therapy, and improve patient outcomes since they regularly encounter patients with upper airway problems.

The Burden of Asthma and Allergic Rhinitis: Epidemiology and Health Care Costs   179

Kunjan B. Patel, James W. Mims, and John D. Clinger

> Allergic rhinitis affects up to 78% of people with asthma, and asthma occurs in 38% of people with allergic rhinitis. Asthma has a prevalence of 8.7% among adults and 6.2% among children and accounts for $50 billion in medical costs and $32 billion in indirect and mortality costs in the United States, respectively. Allergic rhinitis occurs in 5% to 15% of people in the United States. Allergic rhinitis also accounts for a significant health care cost burden, predominantly in terms of indirect costs related to reduced quality of life and presenteeism.

Incorporating Asthma Evaluation into the Otolaryngic Allergy Practice: Presentation and Diagnosis   191

Cecelia Damask and Christine Franzese

> Asthma occurs frequently as a comorbid condition in many patients presenting with common otolaryngology conditions, such as allergic rhinitis and chronic sinusitis with nasal polyps. The classic presentation of asthma includes symptoms of wheezing, shortness of breath, and chest tightness but can include other symptoms such as cough. The diagnosis is made mainly through history, although pulmonary function testing, spirometry, fractional exhaled nitric oxide, and impulse oscillometry may also prove helpful.

Interpretation of Spirometry, Peak Flow, and Provocation Testing for Asthma   201

Sukhmani Boparai and George M. Solomon

> Spirometry plays a crucial role in the diagnosis of asthma. The hallmark spirometry finding of expiratory airflow variability can be demonstrated in several ways including peak airflow and bronchodilator and bronchoprovocation testing. Challenges of overdiagnosis and underdiagnosis underscore the need to consider clinical context while interpreting these tests. A meticulous and multifaceted approach prioritizing objective testing is imperative while diagnosing asthma.

Asthma Management Considerations for the Otolaryngologist: Current Therapies   215

Dhanya Asokumar and Amarbir S. Gill

> Asthma is frequently comorbid with chronic rhinosinusitis. First-line pharmacologic intervention for asthma includes combination-inhaled corticosteroids with a long-acting-β-agonist, preferably formoterol. Although short-acting-β-agonists have historically been used as sole rescue option, studies show that this approach can lead to more asthma-related exacerbations and greater mortality. Similarly, oral corticosteroids should be used sparingly due to their significant adverse effect profile. Nonpharmacological interventions for asthma include counseling on modifiable risk factors, such as smoking, physical activity, occupational exposures, and healthy diets. Management of patients with unified airway disease should incorporate a multidisciplinary team consisting of otolaryngologists and asthma specialists.

Current and Novel Biologic Therapies for Patients with Asthma and Nasal Polyps   225

Hanna K. Mandl, Jessa E. Miller, and Daniel M. Beswick

> A substantial portion of asthma and nasal polyps (NPs) share a common pathogenesis, which includes type 2-mediated inflammation. Distinct endotypes and phenotypes characterizing asthma and chronic rhinosinusitis have been identified. With emerging evidence describing pathophysiology, novel targets for biologic monoclonal antibody treatments have been developed. There are currently six biologic therapies approved by the US Food and Drug Administration to treat asthma, including omalizumab, mepolizumab, reslizumab, benralizumab, dupilumab, and tezepelumab, three of these—omalizumab, mepolizumab, and dupilumab—are also approved for NPs.

Promising New Diagnostic and Treatment Modalities for Allergic Rhinitis: What's Coming Next?   243

Thomas F. Barrett and Lauren T. Roland

> Novel diagnostic tests may help diagnose patients with local allergic rhinitis (AR) when systemic testing is negative or inconclusive. Surgical approaches including septoplasty, inferior turbinate reduction, nasal swell body reduction, and posterior nasal nerve ablation may improve symptoms in patients whose symptoms are refractory to medical therapy, though high-quality evidence is lacking in the AR population. Intralymphatic and epicutaneous immunotherapy have the potential to improve adherence to allergen immunotherapy, though comparisons with current gold standard treatments are lacking and studies reporting long-term

outcomes are needed. Immunomodulatory agents in combination with subcutaneous immunotherapy (SCIT) may improve tolerance of SCIT but reports to date do not demonstrate a clear benefit in symptom alleviation. Future work in these areas may support these options as beneficial for testing and treatment of AR.

Allergy and Asthma Prevalence and Management Across Nasal Polyp Subtypes   253

Kody G. Bolk, Thomas S. Edwards, Sarah K. Wise, and John M. DelGaudio

Allergy and asthma prevalence vary across different subsets of chronic rhinosinusitis with nasal polyposis. In this article, the authors investigate the management of allergy and asthma within populations of patients with aspirin-exacerbated respiratory disease, allergic fungal rhinosinusitis, and central compartment atopic disease. Topical steroids, nasal rinses, and endoscopic sinus surgery are frequently employed in the management of nasal polyposis. Further, other causes of upper and lower airway inflammation like allergy and asthma should be considered in the overall treatment plan in order to optimize outcomes.

Management of Aspirin-Exacerbated Respiratory Disease: What Does the Future Hold?   265

Erin K. O'Brien, Elina Jerschow, and Rohit D. Divekar

Aspirin-exacerbated respiratory disease (AERD) is a subtype of chronic rhinosinusitis with polyps (CRSwNP) and asthma with higher recurrence of nasal polyps after surgery and severe asthma. Patients with CRSwNP and asthma should be screened for AERD by detailed history of aspirin/nonsteroidal anti-inflammatory drug reactions and review of medications that may mask aspirin reaction or directly by aspirin challenge. Treatment of AERD may require more intensive therapy, including endoscopic sinus surgery, daily aspirin therapy, leukotriene modifiers, or biologics.

Update on the Role of Fungus in Allergy, Asthma, and the Unified Airway   279

Brian H. Cameron, Shaina W. Gong, David B. Corry, and Amber U. Luong

The united airway refers to the combined upper and lower airways and their interconnected pathophysiologic relationships. Inflammatory airway diseases (chronic rhinosinusitis, asthma, and so forth) have been linked to fungal species through type 2 immune responses. These type 2 immune responses involve the cytokines interleukin (IL)-4, IL-5, IL-13, and a myriad of other inflammatory processes that lead to a spectrum of diseases from allergic bronchopulmonary mycosis to chronic rhinosinusitis. Historically, these diseases have been managed primarily with corticosteroids but recent revelations in the molecular pathophysiology provide opportunities for more diverse treatment options for patients with uncontrolled disease.

Air Quality, Allergic Rhinitis, and Asthma   293

Abdulrahman Alenezi, Hannan Qureshi, Omar G. Ahmed, and Murugappan Ramanathan Jr.

This review article highlights air pollution as a critical global health concern with emphasis on its effects and role in the development and exacerbation of upper airway and lower airway disease with a focus on allergic rhinitis and asthma. This review underscores the World Health Organization's recognition of air pollution as the biggest environmental threat to human health. It discusses the various components and categories of air pollutants and the evidence-based effects they have on asthma and allergic rhinitis, ranging from pathogenesis to exacerbation of these conditions across various age groups in different geographic locations.

How Does Climate Change Affect the Upper Airway?   309

Jean Kim, Benjamin Zaitchik, and Darryn Waugh

There is mounting evidence that climate change is having a significant influence on exacerbations of airway disease. We herein explore the physical factors of carbon dioxide, temperature increases, and humidity on intensifying allergen and fungal growth, and worsening air quality. The direct influence of these factors on promoting allergic rhinitis, chronic rhinosinusitis, and allergic fungal rhinosinusitis is reviewed.

Allergic Rhinitis and Its Effect on Sleep   319

Jessica M.L. Pagel and Jose L. Mattos

Allergic rhinitis (AR) is associated with increased sleep disturbances in adults and children. Pathogenesis is multifactorial, with nasal obstruction playing a large role. Intranasal corticosteroids, antihistamines, leukotriene inhibitors, and allergen immunotherapy have been demonstrated to relieve self-reported symptoms of sleep impairment. Given the high prevalence of sleep impairment in AR, providers should consider evaluating any patient with AR for sleep disturbances and sleep-disordered breathing.

Molecular Allergology and Component-Resolved Diagnosis in Current Clinical Practice   329

Michael S. Benninger and Gary A. Falcetano

Specific immunoglobulin E immunodiagnostics is becoming a convenient way to identify allergic patients and their specific allergies. These results are comparable to skin testing and may be more accessible for some populations. Each allergen contains thousands of molecules but only a few of these molecules are allergenic to humans. Each allergen has a number of individual components—generally proteins—which have different characteristics that may impact the effects of sensitization. Identification of the specific component allows for differentiation of the true allergies and can help to determine the risk of a significant clinical response.

Eosinophilic Esophagitis: What the Otolaryngologist Needs to Know   343

Nainika Nanda and Dinesh Chhetri

Eosinophilic esophagitis is a male-predominant disease with presentations ranging from nonspecific feeding issues to dysphagia and food impaction. The currently proposed pathophysiology is a combination of genetics, allergens, and epithelial barrier impairment. Diagnosis is reliant on history, endoscopic examination, and biopsy. Recent guidelines recognize the role of concurrent gastroesophageal reflux disease. Treatment is based on 3 paradigms: diet, drugs, and dilation. Drug therapy has historically focused on topical corticosteroids; as of 2022, dupilumab was approved for targeted biologic therapy. Dilation is reserved for symptomatic and anatomic management. As this clinical entity is better understood, additional therapies will hopefully be developed.

OTOLARYNGOLOGIC CLINICS
OF NORTH AMERICA

FORTHCOMING ISSUES

June 2024
Sleep Apnea in Children and Adults
Stacey Ishman, Carol Li, and Reena
Dhanda Patil, *Editors*

August 2024
Dysphagia in Adults and Children
Mausumi Syamal and Eileen Raynor,
Editors

October 2024
Artificial Intelligence in Otolaryngology
Anais Rameau and Matthew G. Crowson,
Editors

RECENT ISSUES

February 2024
Thyroid and Parathyroid Disease
Amy Y. Chen and Michael C. Singer,
Editors

December 2023
Otolaryngologic Trauma
Sydney C. Butts, *Editor*

October 2023
External Ear Disease
Esther X. Vivas and Matthew B. Hanson,
Editors

SERIES OF RELATED INTEREST

Facial Plastic Surgery Clinics
Available at: https://www.facialplastic.theclinics.com/

THE CLINICS ARE AVAILABLE ONLINE!
Access your subscription at:
www.theclinics.com

Foreword

Runny Noses, Postnasal Drip, and Wheezing

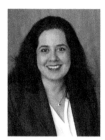

Sujana S. Chandrasekhar, MD, FAAO-HNS, FAOS, FACS
Consulting Editor

In the 1997 movie "As Good As It Gets,"[1] Jack Nicholson's character has obsessive-compulsive disorder and cannot abide the absence of the one waitress who can handle his needs, who is out caring for her wheezing son. He sends a physician to her home who asks Helen Hunt's character if the child has ever been tested for allergies or seen when healthy, and she replies in the negative to both as she produces a diary and tons of medicines that have not worked. To fast forward (and this is a spoiler alert), the child's allergies and asthma, confounded by poor air quality, are managed effectively, and he can return to school and play, the waitress can return to work, and peace once again reigns. I very much appreciate it when movie makers address complex medical issues. Not only does this bring awareness to the public but also it helps physicians and other health care providers appreciate and understand the patient and family's perspectives.

Many aspects of Otolaryngologic illness are cross-cared-for by other specialty providers. Patients who have allergies and asthma seek relief from Otolaryngologists, Allergists, Pulmonologists, and even Gastroenterologists, often managed and overseen by their Primary Care Providers. Our understanding of the Unified Airway, extending from columnar epithelium of the nares to squamous type I alveolar epithelial cells of the lung, continues to evolve. This is because of the varied input from researchers and clinicians from all of these walks of medical life.

In this issue of *Otolaryngologic Clinics of North America*, Drs Daniel Beswick and Sarah Wise have given us a detailed understanding of all aspects of Allergy and Asthma as they should be known by practicing Otolaryngologists. The fifteen articles encompassing this state-of-the-art compilation are each internally complete and together make an even better whole. The articles cover the gamut, from learning details about the Unified Airway to how to incorporate Allergy and some level of Asthma care

Otolaryngol Clin N Am 57 (2024) xiii–xiv
https://doi.org/10.1016/j.otc.2024.01.001
0030-6665/24/© 2024 Published by Elsevier Inc.

into one's Otolaryngology practice to the current and future understanding and treatment of nasal polyps and rhinitis. Still more articles cover Aspirin and respiratory disease, the role of fungus, how allergic rhinitis affects sleep, eosinophilic esophagitis, and getting the diagnosis down to the molecular level. The inclusion of two articles on air quality and climate change is a testament to the important concept that we practice as physicians and other health care providers, and also as citizens of the world.

I hope you enjoy reading this issue of *Otolaryngologic Clinics of North America* as much as I have, and that you also take some time to smell the roses, unless, of course, you are allergic.

Sujana S. Chandrasekhar, MD, FAAO-HNS, FAOS, FACS
Consulting Editor, Otolaryngologic Clinics of North America
President, American Otological Society
Past President, American Academy of Otolaryngology-Head and Neck Surgery
Partner, ENT & Allergy Associates, LLP
Clinical Professor, Department of Otolaryngology-Head and Neck Surgery, Zucker
School of Medicine at Hofstra-Northwell
Clinical Associate Professor, Department of Otolaryngology-Head and Neck Surgery
Icahn School of Medicine at Mount Sinai
18 East 48th Street, 2nd Floor
New York, NY 10017, USA

E-mail address:
ssc@nyotology.com

REFERENCE

1. 'As Good As It Gets'—the doctor's visit. Available at: https://youtu.be/G2WNAQe2Wf0?si=5DcK8cXcBiaZ5tTy. Accessed December 31, 2023.

Preface

Allergy and Asthma in Otolaryngology: Current Management Paradigms

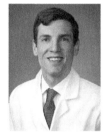 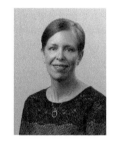

Daniel M. Beswick, MD   Sarah K. Wise, MD
Editors

Allergic and atopic diseases impact the airway from the nares to the alveoli. Otolaryngologists commonly manage these pathologies and are often the primary contact in the health care system for patients with these diseases. This collection includes up-to-date management strategies for allergic rhinitis, rhinosinusitis, and asthma in otolaryngologic settings, including diagnosis, treatment, anticipated future therapies, and associated comorbidities.

In this issue, Hannikainen and colleagues discuss the value of the unified airway model and highlight connections between allergic rhinitis, chronic rhinosinusitis, and asthma. Patel and colleagues review the economic and societal burden of asthma and allergic rhinitis, which together comprise indirect costs estimated to exceed $85 billion annually.

Damask and Franzese discuss the critical points for incorporating asthma diagnosis into an otolaryngologyic allergy practice, including considerations around symptoms, spirometry, fractional exhaled nitric oxide, and impulse oscillometry. Boparai and Solomon provide a detailed review of pulmonary function testing and asthma diagnosis. Asokumar and Gill review the common cormorbid presentation of asthma and chronic rhinosinsuitis and discuss stepwise and escalating use of conventional therapies to optimally manage asthma. Miller and colleagues discuss current and evolving biologic therapies as treatment options for patients with asthma and chronic rhinosinusitis with nasal polyps.

Barrett and Roland review the latest management strategies for allergic rhinitis, including nasal allergen-specific IgE testing, surgical techniques, and burgeoning methods of immunotherapy. Bolk and colleagues discuss the management of asthma

Otolaryngol Clin N Am 57 (2024) xv–xvi
https://doi.org/10.1016/j.otc.2023.12.002
0030-6665/24/© 2023 Published by Elsevier Inc.

and allergy across multiple subtypes of nasal polyp disease, including aspirin-exacerbated respiratory disease, allergic fungal rhinosinusitis, and central compartment atopic disease. O'Brien and colleagues delve into details on optimal diagnostic strategies and upcoming treatments for aspirin-exacerbated respiratory disease. Cameron and colleagues provide a state-of-the-art review on the role of fungus in allergic rhinitis and asthma and describe fungi-mediated airway inflammation.

Alenezi and colleagues present critical information on the adverse effects of air pollutants on upper and lower airway disease. Kim and colleagues review the evidence related to climate change and the increasing prevalence of allergic rhinitis, chronic rhinosinusitis, and allergic fungal rhinosinusitis. Pagel and Mattos discuss the negative impacts of allergic rhinitis on sleep quality and comprehensively discuss medical and surgical therapies for this condition. Benninger and colleagues review component-resolved diagnostic testing and recent developments that facilitate use of this modality. Nanda and Chhetri discuss diagnosis of and management strategies for eosinophilic esophagitis. Overall, this collection of articles provides an up-to-date, accessible, and comprehensive review of these critical components of allergy and asthma for the otolaryngologist.

Daniel M. Beswick, MD
Department of Head and Neck Surgery
University of California, Los Angeles
200 Medical Plaza Drive, Suite 550
Los Angeles, CA 90095, USA

Sarah K. Wise, MD
Department of Otolaryngology–
Head and Neck Surgery
Emory University
550 Peachtree Street, MOT Suite 1135
Atlanta, GA 30030, USA

E-mail addresses:
dbeswick@mednet.ucla.edu (D.M. Beswick)
skmille@emory.edu (S.K. Wise)

Allergic Rhinitis, Rhinosinusitis, and Asthma
Connections Across the Unified Airway

Paavali Hannikainen, BS[a],*, Chase Kahn, MD[b,1],
Elina Toskala, MD, PhD, MBA[b,2]

KEYWORDS

• Allergic rhinitis • Asthma • Unified airway • Inflammation • Shared immunity

KEY POINTS

• Asthma prevalence among patients with rhinitis is estimated to be as high as 40%, and approximately 80% of asthma patients were found to also have concurrent rhinitis.
• Patients who are diagnosed with both rhinitis and asthma typically suffer from a more severe disease that is more difficult and expensive to treat compared to those without both rhinitis and asthma.
• Upper airway and lower airway diseases demonstrate common pathophysiological manifestations making it essential for otolaryngologists to understand the lower airway pathology of allergic disease.
• A comprehensive understanding of the unified airway facilitates early detection and treatment of patients with lower airway disease, further improving patient outcomes.

INTRODUCTION

The connection between allergic inflammatory diseases of the upper and lower airways is well studied in epidemiologic and physiologic research. This relationship is exemplified by the occurrence of upper and lower airway diseases, such as allergic rhinitis (AR), rhinosinusitis, and asthma in the same patients. The term "unified airway" refers to the upper and lower respiratory tracts as a unitary entity consisting of the nose, paranasal sinuses, pharynx, larynx, trachea, bronchi, and alveoli. The unified airway model is predicated on the observation that, upon allergen exposure, the allergic response is not restricted to a single target organ; rather, allergen exposure results in both a local and system-wide effect involving the entire respiratory tract.

[a] Sidney Kimmel Medical College, Thomas Jefferson University, Philadelphia, PA, USA;
[b] Department of Otolaryngology, Thomas Jefferson University, Philadelphia, PA, USA
[1] Present address: 111 South 15th Street P211, Philadelphia, PA 19102.
[2] Present address: 50 South 16th Street, Apartment 4908, Philadelphia, PA 19102.
* Corresponding author. 925 Chestnut Street, Philadelphia, PA 19107.
E-mail address: pah020@students.jefferson.edu

Otolaryngol Clin N Am 57 (2024) 171–178
https://doi.org/10.1016/j.otc.2023.08.009
0030-6665/24/© 2023 Elsevier Inc. All rights reserved.

oto.theclinics.com

Under the unified airway, AR, rhinosinusitis, and asthma are viewed as manifestations of the same disease process.[1]

Due to the close relationship between these upper airway diseases and lower airway pathology, such as asthma and chronic cough, it is essential to understand the lower airway manifestations of allergic disease. In this patient population, the otolaryngologist may be the first practitioner to suspect and diagnose all these diseases. A comprehensive understanding of the unified airway facilitates early identification and treatment of asthma, improving patient outcomes.[2,3]

ALLERGIC RHINITIS

AR is an immunoglobulin E (IgE)-mediated inflammation of the nasal mucosa. AR affects an estimated 400 million individuals worldwide, making it the most prevalent atopic disease, and its prevalence is increasing worldwide.[4] The prevalence of AR in the United States has been estimated to range between 15% and 30% based on physician diagnoses and self-reported nasal symptoms.[5]

AR includes symptoms such as rhinorrhea, nasal obstruction, nasal irritation, sneezing, and postnasal drip. These symptoms are either reversible on their own or with treatment. Allergic Rhinitis and its Impact on Asthma (ARIA) classifies AR symptoms as intermittent when they occur less than 4 days per week or for less than 4 consecutive weeks, and persistent when they occur more than 4 days per week for more than 4 consecutive weeks.[6,7] The majority of individuals with persistent AR experience daily symptoms. AR is moderate/severe when 1 or more of the following symptoms are present: disturbed sleep; impaired daily activities, leisure/sport, education, or employment; or if the patient finds the symptoms bothersome. When none of these symptoms are evident, AR is considered mild. Other types of rhinitis include infectious, occupational, drug-induced, and hormonal; rhinitis can be brought on by irritants, food, or emotions, or it can be atrophic or idiopathic. AR is the most prevalent non-infectious form of rhinitis.[4]

ASTHMA

Asthma is a chronic inflammatory disease characterized by recurrent shortness of breath, wheezing, and chest constriction. The duration and intensity of these symptoms differ with exposure to stimuli. According to the Global Initiative for Asthma (GINA), a history of respiratory symptoms and substantiation of variable expiratory ventilation limitation are required to diagnose asthma.[8]

Based on the frequency and severity of symptoms, prevalence of nighttime symptoms, and spirometry findings, asthma can be classified as mild intermittent, mild persistent, moderate persistent, or severe persistent. The GINA guidelines recommend treating asthma using a step-by-step approach with treatment modifications based on the requirements of the individual patient. Important new adjustments to the guidelines in 2022 recommend low-dose inhaled corticosteroid in combination with formoterol as a reliever medication, moving away from short-acting beta-2 agonists like albuterol.[8] This has been shown to improve asthma control and reduce exacerbations.[9]

THE UNIFIED AIRWAY MODEL

The term "unified airway" refers to the view of the upper and lower airways as a singular unit, made up of the nostrils, paranasal sinuses, pharynx, larynx, trachea, bronchi, and pulmonary alveoli. Local inflammatory processes and a systemic response caused by the migration of proinflammatory mediators into the circulatory system occur in response to allergen exposure. Under this paradigm, upper and lower airway diseases, such as rhinitis and asthma, can be viewed as manifestations of a single disease.[1]

Edema and vasodilation result from inflammation of the nasal mucosa, whereas inflammation of the bronchial mucosa causes smooth muscle contraction.[10] Studies have shown that antigen stimulation at a single respiratory site induces an inflammatory response at distal and distinct respiratory sites. Several studies have revealed this pathophysiologic connection, helping explain the unified airway model.[11–13]

Unified airway diseases have clinical implications. Studies examining prescription data revealed that patients with asthma and AR had a higher prescription medication utilization rate than those with asthma alone.[2] Several studies have demonstrated that the treatment of rhinitis in asthmatic patients reduces lower airway symptoms, emergency department visits, and hospitalizations.[14–16]

ALLERGIC RHINITIS AND ASTHMA

There is a distinct epidemiologic connection between AR and asthma, and the 2 conditions frequently coexist in the same patients. Asthma affects approximately 8% of the population in the United States[17]; however, the prevalence of asthma in patients with AR has been estimated to be as high as 40%. In addition, 30% of patients with AR who do not have asthma exhibit bronchial hyperreactivity in response to methacholine or histamine challenge.[10] In contrast, over 80% of asthmatic individuals have AR.[18,19]

Not only is there a strong correlation between AR and asthma, but AR is also considered an independent risk factor for the development of asthma in the future. Multiple long-term studies have shown that patients with AR are 3 times more likely to develop asthma than those without rhinitis.[20–22] The temporal connection between AR and asthma has also been investigated. AR typically precedes or co-occurs with the development of asthma with approximately 65% of those with AR and asthma developed rhinitis symptoms prior to or concurrently with the onset of lower airway symptoms.[21]

Patients with both rhinitis and asthma typically suffer from a more severe disease that is more difficult and expensive to treat.[23,24] Large population-based investigations have demonstrated a correlation between the 2 diseases' severity.[25–27] Patients with concomitant AR have not only more asthma-related hospitalizations and physician visits, those with AR also fill significantly more prescriptions for asthma treatment and incur higher asthma-related drug costs.[26]

CHRONIC RHINOSINUSITIS AND ASTHMA

By definition, chronic rhinosinusitis (CRS) is described as an inflammation of the nose and paranasal sinuses that lasts at least 12 weeks. CRS is characterized by anterior or posterior rhinorrhea, nasal obstruction, facial pain and/or pressure, and alterations in the sense of scent.[28] CRS affects an estimated 31 million patients annually in the United States, and its prevalence continues to rise. CRS is a significant health care issue that results in frequent doctor visits, substantial medication-related costs, and indirect costs incurred by the patient.[29]

A correlation between CRS and asthma has been observed on an epidemiologic level. The prevalence of asthma in the general population of the United States is approximately 8%, while it is estimated to be at least 20% among patients with CRS. Approximately 40% of patients with CRS who ultimately undergo functional endoscopic sinus surgery develop asthma. In CRS patients with nasal polyps, the prevalence is even greater.[30]

Patients with asthma and concurrent CRS have a more severe disease that requires more aggressive treatment.[31] The coexistence of CRS and asthma has detrimental effects on patient outcomes, including pulmonary function and quality of life, compared to asthma patients alone.[32] Frequent asthma exacerbations are substantially associated with severe sinonasal disease.

Recent studies have focused on understanding the role of T lymphocytes of types 1, 2, and 3 (termed T1, T2, and T3) endotypes in CRS, which drive inflammatory patterns in tissues. The primary cytokine(s) of T1 endotype is interferon-gamma, T2 endotype are interleukin-4 (IL-4), IL-5, and IL-13, and T3 endotype is IL-17. Specifically, T2 inflammation with elevation of T2 cytokines and eosinophil proteins is found in CRS patients with asthma.[33,34] One study found that T2 endotype in patients with CRS is associated with asthma comorbidity, nasal polyposis, smell loss, and allergic mucin.[35] Furthermore, another study of Chinese patients with CRS found elevated T2 inflammation and comorbid asthma having the poorest outcomes and most severe clinical manifestation.[36]

PATHOPHYSIOLOGY

Several proposed mechanisms explain the relationship between upper and lower airway inflammation. There is accumulating evidence supporting the shared immunity pathophysiologic mechanism as an explanation for the common inflammatory processes observed in the upper and lower respiratory tracts in response to allergen exposure.[37]

In addition, recent genetic studies have begun to reveal the genetic variations in upper and lower airway disease, with genetic factors accounting for up to 90% of AR and 25% to 80% of asthma risk. The identified genes regulate cytokine signaling, tissue remodeling, the metabolism of arachidonic acid, innate immunity, and other proinflammatory mechanisms.[38] However, these diseases have multiple risk alleles and a strong relationship between environmental exposures and disease development.

Role of Nasal Breathing

The nostril filters, warms, and humidifies inhaled air prior to its entry into the lower airway. One proposed mechanism to explain the observed association between nasal inflammation and lower airway disease proposes that nasal dysfunction resulting from AR reduces a person's ability to breathe through the nose, forcing mouth-breathing and resulting in the loss of the nasal protective mechanism.

Aspiration of Nasal Discharge

Aspiration of nasal contents into the tracheobronchial tree has been proposed as a mechanism for the physiologic connection between the upper and lower airways. Multiple studies conducted to ascertain the effect of aspiration of nasal contents on bronchial reactivity have yielded contradictory findings.[18]

Nasobronchial Reflex

A third mechanism postulated to explain the relationship between the upper and lower airways suggests that the responsible mechanism is a nasobronchial reflex, in which contaminants in the nostril trigger bronchospasm and the development of asthma via neural signaling. Stimulation of the reflex by irritation of the nasal mucosa results in afferent signaling to the central nervous system along the trigeminal nerve. In response to vagus nerve efferent signaling, smooth muscle contraction and bronchoconstriction occur. This mechanism has been extensively investigated, but the significance of this reflex is still debatable.

Shared Immunity

Upper and lower airways can be viewed as a singular, integrated organ affected by a shared inflammatory process. Local and systemic reactions occur in response to allergen exposure, resulting in upper and lower airway manifestations of allergic disease. Several histologic characteristics are shared by the upper and lower respiratory tracts, including pseudostratified ciliated columnar epithelium, goblet cells, fibroblasts, inflammatory cells, and nerves. However, there are structural distinctions between the upper and lower airways, which result in the unique physical manifestations of allergic inflammation at each respiratory site. Large subepithelial capillary and arterial networks, as well as venous cavernous sinuses, characterize the upper airway. Therefore, vasodilation and edema result from sinonasal inflammation, causing nasal congestion and rhinorrhea. In the presence of comparable inflammatory factors, the presence of smooth muscle causes contraction and bronchial hyperresponsiveness in the lower airway. Consequently, the upper and lower airways are subject to a shared inflammatory process that manifests variably at various respiratory sites.

IgE overproduction in response to common environmental allergens, such as pollens, fungi, dust mites, and animal debris, causes AR and atopic asthma.[4] Both disease processes are dependent on initial allergen exposure, which results in a cascade of events leading to the isotype transition from IgM, the first class of Ig presented on B-cells, to IgE, the Ig primarily responsible for the allergic response. IgE generated by B-cells attaches with high affinity to FcR1 on the membranes of mast cells and basophils. Upon subsequent exposure to the previously sensitized antigen, these cells are activated via the FcR1, resulting in the degranulation of mast cells and basophils. The release of mediators such as histamine and leukotrienes causes an immediate hypersensitivity response. This instantaneous response includes sneezing, pruritus, rhinorrhea, coughing, and dyspnea. Eosinophils and basophils, which are recruited by Th2 cells in response to the cytokines IL-4 and IL-5, play a crucial role in the perpetuation of the allergic response, which leads to a chronic inflammatory state.

Several significant investigations have demonstrated the pathophysiological link between the upper and lower airways via systemic circulation. Segmental bronchial provocation (SBP) in non-asthmatic patients with AR has been shown to induce peripheral blood eosinophilia and allergic inflammation at distant respiratory sites.[11] In a subsequent study, in non-asthmatic patients with AR, SBP resulted in a decrease in nasal mucosal mast cells owing to enhanced degranulation. After segmental bronchial provocation, there was a decrease in basophils in the peripheral bloodstream and an increase in basophils in the nasal and bronchial mucosa, providing some evidence for basophil migration from the blood into the nasal and bronchial mucosa.[12] In contrast, nasal provocation has been shown to increase adhesion molecules (ICAM-1, VCAM-1, and E-selectin) and eosinophils in the upper and lower airways.[13]

SUMMARY

Upper and lower inflammatory diseases are closely related and coexist frequently in the same patients. There are significant epidemiologic links between AR and asthma, and AR is a known, independent risk factor for the development of asthma in the future. In addition, the development of AR tends to precede or coincide with the onset of asthma. Similarly, there is a correlation between CRS and asthma, and it has been demonstrated that treating CRS effectively improves asthma outcomes. Therefore, otolaryngologists are in a unique position to identify not only individuals with undiagnosed asthma, but also those at risk for the development of lower airway disease who may benefit from preventive treatment strategies.

CLINICS CARE POINTS

- Due to the close relationship between upper airway diseases (eg, AR, CRS) and lower airway pathology (eg, asthma, chronic cough), it is essential to understand the lower airway manifestations of allergic disease.
- Studies have demonstrated that the treatment of upper airway inflammation in asthmatic patients reduces lower airway symptoms, emergency department visits, and hospitalizations.
- There have been multiple postulated mechanisms to explain the relationship between upper and lower airway diseases including the effect of nasal defense mechanism, aspiration of nasal contents, and nasobronchial reflex; however, multiple studies have yielded contradictory findings.
- There is pathophysiologic support for the shared immunity mechanism underlying the observation of the unified airway model linking upper and lower inflammatory diseases.
- Otolaryngologists can play a crucial role to help identify individuals who are at risk of developing lower respiratory inflammatory disease and may prevent further comorbidities seen in these populations with early preventive treatment strategies.

DISCLOSURE

E. Toskala – GSK: speakers' bureau, research funding, consultant; Aerin: consultant; Optinose: research funding; Medtronic: consultant.

REFERENCES

1. Passalacqua G, Ciprandi G, Canonica GW. United airways disease: therapeutic aspects. Thorax, 55. BMJ Publishing Group Ltd; 2000. p. S26–7.
2. Pillsbury HC, Krouse JH, Marple BF, et al. The impact/role of asthma in otolaryngology. Otolaryngol Head Neck Surg 2007;136(1):157.
3. Shtraks JP, Toskala E. Manifestations of inhalant allergies beyond the nose. Otolaryngol Clin 2017;50(6):1051–64.
4. Pawankar R. Allergic diseases and asthma: a global public health concern and a call to action. World Allergy Organ J 2014;7(1):1–3.
5. Greiner AN, Hellings PW, Rotiroti G, et al. Allergic rhinitis. Lancet 2011;378(9809): 2112–22.
6. Brożek JL, Bousquet J, Baena-Cagnani CE, et al. Allergic rhinitis and its impact on asthma (ARIA) guidelines: 2010 revision. J Allergy Clin Immunol 2010;126(3): 466–76.
7. Brożek JL, Bousquet J, Agache I, et al. Allergic rhinitis and its impact on asthma (ARIA) guidelines—2016 revision. J Allergy Clin Immunol 2017;140(4):950–8.
8. Global Initiative for Asthma. 2022 GINA Main Report - Global Initiative for Asthma.; 2022. https://ginasthma.org/gina-reports/. Accessed March 15, 2023.
9. Sobieraj DM, Weeda ER, Nguyen E, et al. Association of inhaled corticosteroids and long-acting β-agonists as controller and quick relief therapy with

exacerbations and symptom control in persistent asthma: a systematic review and meta-analysis. JAMA 2018;319(14):1485–96.

10. Giavina-Bianchi P, Vivolo Aun M, Takejima P, et al. United airway disease: current perspectives. J Asthma Allergy 2016;9:93–100.

11. Braunstahl GJ, Kleinjan A, Overbeek SE, et al. Segmental bronchial provocation induces nasal inflammation in allergic rhinitis patients. Am J Respir Crit Care Med 2000;161(6):2051–7.

12. Braunstahl G-J, Overbeek SE, Fokkens WJ, et al. Segmental bronchoprovocation in allergic rhinitis patients affects mast cell and basophil numbers in nasal and bronchial mucosa. Am J Respir Crit Care Med 2001;164(5):858–65.

13. Braunstahl GJ, Overbeek SE, KleinJan A, et al. Nasal allergen provocation induces adhesion molecule expression and tissue eosinophilia in upper and lower airways. J Allergy Clin Immunol 2001;107(3):469–76.

14. Stelmach R, Nunes MDPT, Ribeiro M, et al. Effect of treating allergic rhinitis with corticosteroids in patients with mild-to-moderate persistent asthma. Chest 2005; 128(5):3140–7.

15. Watson WTA, Becker AB, Simons FER. Treatment of allergic rhinitis with intranasal corticosteroids in patients with mild asthma: effect on lower airway responsiveness. J Allergy Clin Immunol 1993;91(1 PART 1):97–101.

16. Fuhlbrigge AL, Adams RJ. The effect of treatment of allergic rhinitis on asthma morbidity, including emergency department visits. Curr Opin Allergy Clin Immunol 2003;3(1):29–32.

17. Center for Disease Control and Preventions (CDC). Most Recent National Asthma Data. Asthma Data Statistics and Surveilance. https://www.cdc.gov/asthma/most_recent_national_asthma_data.htm. Published 2022. Accessed March 15, 2023.

18. Corren J. Allergic rhinitis and asthma: How important is the link? J Allergy Clin Immunol 1997;99(2):S781–6.

19. Custovic A, Simpson A. The role of inhalant allergens in allergic airways disease. J Investig Allergol Clin Immunol 2012;22(6):393–401.

20. Guerra S, Sherrill DL, Martinez FD, et al. Rhinitis as an independent risk factor for adult-onset asthma. J Allergy Clin Immunol 2002;109(3):419–25.

21. Settipane RJ, Hagy GW, Settipane GA. Long-term risk factors for developing asthma and allergic rhinitis: A 23- year follow-up study of college students. Allergy Proc 1994;15(1):21–5.

22. Settipane RJ. Co-existence of asthma and allergic rhinitis: A 23-year follow-up study of college students. Allergy Asthma Proc 1998;19(4):185–8.

23. Halpern MT, Schmier JK, Richner R, et al. Allergic rhinitis: a potential cause of increased asthma medication use, costs, and morbidity. J Asthma 2004;41(1): 117–26.

24. Antonicelli L, Micucci C, Voltolini S, et al. Relationship between ARIA classification and drug treatment in allergic rhinitis and asthma. Allergy Eur J Allergy Clin Immunol 2007;62(9):1064–70.

25. Thomas M, Kocevar VS, Zhang Q, et al. Asthma-related health care resource use among asthmatic children with and without concomitant allergic rhinitis. Pediatrics 2005;115(1):129–34.

26. Price D, Zhang Q, Kocevar VS, et al. Effect of a concomitant diagnosis of allergic rhinitis on asthma-related health care use by adults. Clin Exp Allergy 2005;35(3): 282–7.

27. Ohta K, Bousquet PJ, Aizawa H, et al. Prevalence and impact of rhinitis in asthma. SACRA, a cross-sectional nation-wide study in Japan. Allergy Eur J Allergy Clin Immunol 2011;66(10):1287–95.

28. Yang J, Finke JC, Yang J, et al. Early risk prognosis of free-flap transplant failure by quantitation of the macrophage colony-stimulating factor in patient plasma using 2-dimensional liquid-chromatography multiple reaction monitoring-mass spectrometry. Med (United States) 2016;95(39).

29. Meltzer EO, Hamilos DL, Hadley JA, et al. Rhinosinusitis: establishing definitions for clinical research and patient care. J Allergy Clin Immunol 2004;114(6):155–212.

30. Jani AL, Hamilos DL. Current thinking on the relationship between rhinosinusitis and asthma. J Asthma 2005;42(1):1–7.

31. Stachler RJ. Comorbidities of asthma and the unified airway. Int Forum Allergy Rhinol 2015;5(S1):S17–22.

32. Ek A, Middelveld RJM, Bertilsson H, et al. Chronic rhinosinusitis in asthma is a negative predictor of quality of life: Results from the Swedish GA2LEN survey. Allergy Eur J Allergy Clin Immunol 2013;68(10):1314–21.

33. Zhang N, Van Zele T, Perez-Novo C, et al. Different types of T-effector cells orchestrate mucosal inflammation in chronic sinus disease. J Allergy Clin Immunol 2008;122(5):961–8.

34. Wen W, Liu W, Zhang L, et al. Increased neutrophilia in nasal polyps reduces the response to oral corticosteroid therapy. J Allergy Clin Immunol 2012;129(6):1522–8.

35. Stevens WW, Peters AT, Tan BK, et al. Associations between inflammatory endotypes and clinical presentations in chronic rhinosinusitis. J Allergy Clin Immunol Pract 2019;7(8):2812–20.

36. Liao B, Liu J, Li Z, et al. Multidimensional endotypes of chronic rhinosinusitis and their association with treatment outcomes. Allergy 2018;73(7):1459–69.

37. Krouse JH. The unified airway—conceptual framework. Otolaryngol Clin 2008;41(2):257–66.

38. Brar T, Marino MJ, Lal D. Unified airway disease: genetics and epigenetics. Otolaryngol Clin 2023;56(1):23–38.

The Burden of Asthma and Allergic Rhinitis
Epidemiology and Health Care Costs

Kunjan B. Patel, MD, James W. Mims, MD*, John D. Clinger, MD

KEYWORDS

• Asthma • Allergic rhinitis • Epidemiology • Cost • Prevalence • Unified airway

KEY POINTS

• Asthma and allergic rhinitis (AR) are often comorbid. AR is an independent risk factor for developing asthma.
• Asthma affects approximately 8.7% of adults and 6.2% of children in the United States.
• Symptoms of AR are common, reported by up to 25% of patients in the United States. Symptoms can be nonspecific, however, and many patients report symptoms without positive allergen testing. Therefore, reported AR prevalence varies, estimated to be between 5% and 15% in the United States.
• Asthma accounts for significant direct and indirect health care costs, estimated to be over $80 billion per year.
• AR also accounts for significant health care costs, predominantly in terms of indirect costs related to reduced quality of life, estimated to be approximately $5 billion per year.

THE UNIFIED AIRWAY: HOW ARE ASTHMA AND ALLERGIC RHINITIS RELATED?

Asthma and allergic rhinitis (AR) are 2 commonly diagnosed medical conditions in the United States. Although affecting different portions of the airway, the unified airway model suggests the 2 conditions are interconnected. These interconnections are defined in many ways, including similarities in histology, type 2 inflammatory mediators,[1] and resulting methods of management.[2,3] Incidence studies have supported this model,[2,4] demonstrating presence of AR in 78% of people with asthma and presence of asthma in 38% of people with AR. AR and asthma are also comorbid, with history of AR shown in meta-analyses to be strongly associated with incidence of asthma.[5–8] Perennial AR is noted to be an independent risk factor for the development of asthma,[3,8–10] and patients with perennial AR also appear to have more frequent asthma exacerbations.[11–13] As a result, studying these interrelated conditions together may provide utility in understanding these common, treatable diseases.

Department of Otolaryngology, Wake Forest School of Medicine, Winston-Salem, NC, USA
* Corresponding author. Medical Center Boulevard, Winston-Salem, NC 27157.
E-mail address: wmims@wakehealth.edu

Otolaryngol Clin N Am 57 (2024) 179–189
https://doi.org/10.1016/j.otc.2023.09.007
0030-6665/24/© 2023 Elsevier Inc. All rights reserved.

ASTHMA: DEFINITION

Asthma is an obstructive pulmonary disorder with exacerbations defined by the 1991, 1997, and 2007 National Institutes of Health Guidelines on Asthma.[14,15] It is characterized as a chronic inflammatory disorder, with distinct symptoms of shortness of breath, cough, chest tightness, and/or wheezing. It is a heterogenous disorder and refers to symptoms and physiology, rather than a cause, which can originate from a variety of gene-environment interactions.[16] Consequently, several classification systems exist, including groups based on biomarkers and endotypes, but the inflammatory pathway most often stems from a T helper (Th2) dominant process.[17] One endotype, allergic asthma, deserves specific attention due to distinct pathophysiologic overlap with AR.

Allergic asthma, typically begins in childhood and is characterized by hypersensitivity to allergens triggering exacerbations. It accounts for approximately 50% of childhood asthma[18,19] and requires positivity to skin prick test or specific immunoglobulin E (sIgE). It appears to be associated with milder disease compared to nonallergic asthma. Despite these distinctions, the Th2 mechanism of airway inflammation is still seen in most nonallergic asthma and allergic asthma.[17]

ASTHMA: EPIDEMIOLOGY

Asthma is a frequently diagnosed condition. Globally, the prevalence of asthma is estimated to be approximately 11.5% based on population studies. Prevalence appears to be highest in the African region (13.2%) and lowest in the Americas (10.0%), though data vary by country.[20] In the United States, overall prevalence also varies by state but is increasing slowly overall. In 2022, the percentage of adults with asthma was 8.7%, which had increased from 8% in 2019, according to the Centers for Disease Control (CDC) household interview data. Prevalence of asthma is lower in children, with 6.2% of US children having asthma. The prevalence of asthma has increased slightly with 7.4% of the overall population reporting a diagnosis of asthma in 2000, compared to 7.8% (~25 million) in 2020. Prevalence of asthma varies by state, ranging from 7.3% of population in Florida to 12.4% in West Virginia (2021). Women are more likely to have asthma (8.9%) compared to men (6.5%). Boys (7.3%) are more likely to have asthma than girls (5.6%) (**Fig. 1**). When considering racial differences, African American children have the highest prevalence (11%), and Asians have the lowest prevalence (3.5%). People with asthma are more likely to be younger and have lower socioeconomic status (10.4% below 100% of the poverty threshold compared to 6.8% above 450% of the poverty threshold).

Among patients who have asthma in the United States, 39.6% of adults and 38.7% of children had an asthma exacerbation/attack in the past year. Overall, asthma attack prevalence is decreasing, with 56% of all people diagnosed with asthma reporting an attack in 2001 compared to 40.7% in 2021 (**Fig. 2**). Asthma is the third leading cause of hospitalization among children younger than age 15, but the hospitalization rate is also decreasing (13/10,000 in 2010 compared to 5/10,000 in 2019). In 2021, there were 3517 deaths caused by asthma, with 145 child mortalities, which have both been relatively stable.

ASTHMA: HEALTH CARE COSTS

Asthma is associated with significant costs, both direct and indirect. Direct costs refer to costs resulting from the medical management of the disease. Indirect costs refer to other collateral losses such as lost wages and productivity.

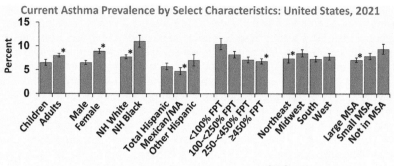

Current Asthma Prevalence by Select Characteristics: United States, 2021

*Reference group

Fig. 1. Asthma prevalence in the United States by select characteristics, 2021. Current asthma prevalence was higher among adults, females, NH Black persons, other Hispanic persons, household income<100% FPT or 100 to<250% FPT, and persons living in small MSA and not in MSAs compared with the corresponding reference groups. Current asthma prevalence did not differ by region. FPT, federal poverty threshold; MA, Mexican-American; MSA, metropolitan statistical area; NH, non-hispanic.*Reference group. (*Data from* CDC, available free of charge: https://www.cdc.gov/asthma/asthmadata.htm. Figure From CDC: https://www.cdc.gov/asthma/Asthma-Prevalence-US-2023-508.pdf. Accessed August 1, 2023.)

A comprehensive study conducted by the CDC and published in 2018[21] examined the medical costs due to asthma from 2008 to 2013 using the Medical Expenditure Panel Survey (MEPS). The MEPS represents a large, nationally representative survey which collects data on demographics and health care use, expenditure, and insurance. The MEPS also gathers data regarding indirect costs based on missed school and work data. It is based on survey data of 214,000 representative patients over 6 years (2008–2013), with an average of 35,000 respondents per year. These respondents included patients with asthma and without asthma, with an asthma prevalence of 4% to 5%. Average costs were compared between these groups, and additional information was obtained from medical providers. Total costs were reported in 2015

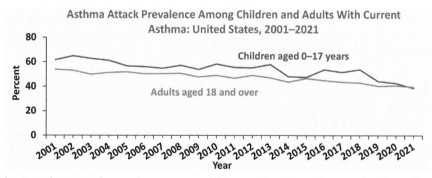

Asthma Attack Prevalence Among Children and Adults With Current Asthma: United States, 2001–2021

Fig. 2. Asthma attack prevalence among children and adults with current asthma. From 2001 to 2021, the percent of children and adults with current asthma who had at least 1 asthma attack in the previous 12 months declined. For children, asthma attacks declined from 61.7% of children with asthma in 2001 to 38.7% in 2021. For adults, asthma attacks declined from 53.8% of adults with asthma in 2001 to 39.6% in 2021. (*Data from* CDC, available free of charge: https://www.cdc.gov/asthma/asthmadata.htm. Figure from CDC: https://www.cdc.gov/asthma/Asthma-Prevalence-US-2023-508.pdf. Accessed August 1, 2023.)

Consumer Price Index–adjusted dollars and were as follows: Annual per-person incremental cost associated with asthma was $3266 more than patients without asthma, with greater than 50% attributable to prescription medication. The cost was $176 for outpatient visits and $105 for emergency room visits. Asthma was responsible for $3 billion in indirect costs (missed work and school days) and $79 billion in medical costs and mortality-related costs. On average, asthma was responsible for 1.8 missed workdays and 2.3 missed school days per person per year. Of note, these costs are likely to under-represent the true cost of asthma as the survey only accounted for "treated" asthma—that is, patients with at least one treatment encounter related to asthma. Over 30% of patients with current asthma did not have an asthma-related encounter with a medical provider or pharmacy. Other indirect costs such as transportation, time lost, and presenteeism were also not accounted.

These costs are anticipated to increase over the next 20 years,[21] with a probabilistic model calculated in 2019 based on state-specific population growth and asthma prevalence trends predicting an estimated $300 billion in direct costs and up to $900 billion in indirect costs in 2039. Overall, asthma continues to be a major contributor to the health care cost burden in the United States. Worldwide costs are difficult to estimate given the variability among health care systems.

ALLERGIC RHINITIS: DEFINITION

AR is one of the most common conditions encountered by otolaryngologists. A commonly accepted definition encapsulates the condition as an immunoglobulin E(IgE)-mediated, type 1 hypersensitivity reaction in the nasal mucosa induced after allergen exposure in a sensitized individual.[22] The IgE-mediated inflammatory response results in a combination of symptoms, which may include sneezing, nasal itching, nasal obstruction, or rhinorrhea.[23,24]

Diagnosis of AR is often made on history and physical examination, but symptoms may not distinguish AR from other causes.[25] Allergy testing, therefore, can be performed to support the diagnosis. Unfortunately, it is common to have test-positive sensitization without allergy symptoms and vice versa, which complicates the definitive diagnosis of AR.

Several subtypes of AR also exist with varying effects on quality of life. The Allergic Rhinitis and its Impact on Asthma initiative organizes AR by cause and timing.[22] The major subtypes included "intermittent" and "persistent." Persistent is defined as having symptoms for more than 4 days per week for more than 4 consecutive weeks, but most classified as persistent have daily symptoms.

AR can also be categorized by severity: "mild" and "moderate/severe."[22] The criteria for "moderate/severe" are listed in **Box 1**. In the absence of any criteria qualifying AR as moderate/severe, AR is categorized as mild. In general, AR classification severity is subjective. Objective allergy test results (wheal size or sIgE level) do not necessarily correlate with symptom severity.[26,27] Given additional confounders such as varying levels of air pollution, multiple triggers, or variability in allergen exposures, studies on the burden and epidemiology of AR may demonstrate marked variability.[28–31]

ALLERGIC RHINITIS: EPIDEMIOLOGY

Several methods have attempted to shed light on the epidemiology of AR. Estimates of prevalence can vary widely based on geography, type of study, and definition of AR used, with reported prevalence between 5% and 50%.[28–31]

One large Swiss study[31] in adults examined the relationship between symptoms and allergy testing in patients who did not self-select as allergic. The SAPALDIA (Swiss

---

Box 1
Determination of severity of allergic rhinitis based on Allergic Rhinitis and its Impact on Asthma 2008 Guidelines

Moderate/severe*

Sleep disturbance

Impairment of daily activities, leisure and/or sport

Impairment of school or work

Troublesome symptoms

*Presence of one or more.

**Mild allergic rhinitis means none of these are present.

Data from Bousquet J, Khaltaev N, Cruz AA, et al. Allergic Rhinitis and its Impact on Asthma (ARIA) 2008 update (in collaboration with the World Health Organization, GA(2)LEN and AllerGen). Allergy. Apr 2008;63 Suppl 86:8-160. doi:10.1111/j.1398-9995.2007.01620.x

---

Study on Air Pollution and Lung Disease in Adults) determined prevalence of AR based on standardized questions and IgE and skin prick testing among Swiss adults. Overall, although 28.9% of patients had a positive allergen-sIgE test and 23% had at least 1 positive skin prick test, only 16.3% of patients reported they suffered from AR or symptoms of AR over the past year. Of the 16.3% of patients with positive symptoms, 77.1% and 68.4% demonstrated positive sIgE and skin prick tests, respectively. These results demonstrate that symptom positivity alone or test positivity alone does not indicate AR diagnosis or clinically meaningful AR severity. The estimated prevalence of AR combining symptoms and allergy tests, therefore, was 11.1% to 12.3% (**Table 1**).

A study in the United States based on the National Health and Nutrition Examination Surveys (NHANES)[30,32] demonstrated that 24% of patients report diagnosis of AR or "hay fever" (term used by NHANES), but 43.7% of all responders had a positive IgE. Among patients reporting symptom positivity, only 74.4% of the "hay fever" and 57.9% of the allergies group had positive sIgE to at least 1 allergen. The estimated prevalence of AR, combining symptoms and allergy tests, was therefore 13.6% (see **Table 1**).

More recent epidemiologic studies conducted in Korea,[33,34] the Netherlands,[34,35] and China[35] bolster these findings and further illustrate the difficulty to definitively characterize the epidemiology of AR, but overall noting the prevalence of AR and sIgE positivity between 5% to 15%. Time of year and study location,[35] given the intermittent nature of some symptoms and the presence of allergens, may also affect results.

Prevalence of AR in the pediatric populations has also been studied. Most studies are cross-sectional, including some of the largest studies. The International Study of Asthma and Allergies in Childhood (ISAAC) is among these studies.[36–39] Questionnaire data on 54,178 children and skin prick testing in 31,759 children showed varying international prevalence across sites in ISAAC phase II studies. Symptom prevalence varied from 1.5% in Ecuador to 24% in Spain, and skin prick test positivity varied from 0.1% in Ghana to 45.2% in Hong Kong.[39] In phases I and III of the ISAAC studies, which depended only on symptom questionnaires, the international prevalence of AR was 8.5% for 6 to 7-year-olds, rising to 14.6% among 13 to 14-year-olds. In the United States, rhinoconjunctivitis symptoms also increased from 13.4% to 19.1% between 6 and 13 to 14-year-olds, respectively. However, as noted earlier, symptoms do not always diagnose AR. A Swedish study in 2009[40] compared a cohort's skin prick tests at ages 7 to 8 and again 10 years later and found an increase from 20.6% to

Table 1
Comparisons of large epidemiologic studies on allergic rhinitis

	SAPALDIA	NHANES II	NHANES III	NHANES 2005–2006
Study size	n = 8329	n = 7230	n = 10,508	n = 7398
Ages	18–60 y	6–59 y	6–59 y	6 y and older
Study location	Switzerland	United States	United States	United States
Questionnaire/Interview				
CAR	16.3%			
CA				23.5%
CHF		5.8%[a,b]	9.7%[a,c]	6.6%
CR				34.2%
Allergy Tests				
sIgE	28.9%			43.2%
SPT	23%	21.8% (6 allergens)	53.9% (10 allergens)	
Positive Survey & Test				
CAR and +SPT	11.1%			
CAR and +sIgE	12.6%			
CA and + sIgE				13.6%
CHF and+ sIgE		Not available	Not available	4.9%
CR and +sIgE				12.8%

Abbreviations: CA, current allergies; CAR, current allergic rhinitis; CHF, current hay fever; CR, current rhinitis; n, number; NHANES, National Health and Nutrition Examination Surveys; SAPALDIA, Swiss Study on Air Pollution and Lung Disease in Adults; sIgE, specific immunoglobulin E; SPT, skin prick test; y, years.
  [a] NHANES II and III—interview and allergy testing on different populations.
  [b] www.cdc.gov/nchs/data/nhanesii/5020.pdf (assessed June 22, 2014).
  [c] ftp://ftp.cdc.gov/pub/Health_Statistics/NCHS/nhanes/nhanes3/1A/ADULT-acc.pdf (accessed June 22, 2014).
  From: Mims JW. Epidemiology of allergic rhinitis. Int Forum Allergy Rhinol. Sep 2014;4 Suppl 2:S18-20. https://doi.org/10.1002/alr.21385 [with permission].

29.9% ($P < .001$) in those with at least 1 positive test. However, the prevalence of rhinitis symptoms in the same subjects only increased from 14.5% to 15.1%. Nonetheless, based on the aforementioned literature, according to both AR symptoms and objective testing, it appears that the prevalence of AR in children increases with age into the teenage years.

Characteristics of certain cohorts make the assessment of AR particularly challenging in those populations. For example, assessing AR prevalence in the preschool age group is difficult due to the ubiquity of viral rhinitis. AR is not thought to be common among children younger than 1 year due to the ongoing development of the immune system. On the other hand, assessing AR in older adults is complicated by the increased prevalence of chronic nonallergic rhinitis and debate regarding possible allergic senescence.

In general, based on these studies, some conclusions about the epidemiology and diagnosis of AR can be made.

1. A substantial percentage of patients with self-reported AR symptoms do not demonstrate positive skin or IgE testing. Self-reported symptoms, therefore, may overpredict AR.

2. Allergy testing in the absence of clinical history can lead to overdiagnosis of AR.
3. AR is a heterogenous disease and can be difficult to diagnose. Therefore, epidemiologic studies are difficult to conduct, and a definitive diagnosis of AR can be difficult to determine.
4. AR diagnoses in preschool age groups and older adults are clinically difficult to determine due to prevalence of viral and nonallergic rhinitis, respectively.
5. Overall, based on both US and European population studies, history and objective testing resulted in AR prevalence of 10% to 15%. However, international studies in children found geographic variation of 0.1% to 45%, implying significant geographic variability.

ALLERGIC RHINITIS: HEALTH CARE COSTS

The difficulty in delineating the epidemiology of AR translates as imprecision in accurately determining its health care costs. In the United States, AR ranks within the top 5 conditions based on total costs, with direct costs exceeding $4.5 billion per year.[41,42] Among direct costs, medication expense,[43,44] estimated to be up to 2 billion US dollars, makes up most of the direct costs since AR generally does not lead to hospitalizations and emergency department visits. However, medication costs appear to be decreasing. This is hypothesized to be due to many medications transitioning to over-the-counter purchasing options where costs are not tracked as easily.[44] On average, AR patients had annual costs of $218 for clinic related visits and $111 for medications based on national insurance claims analysis.[43] A MEPS analysis estimated mean prescription expenditure at $131 based on data from 1996.[45] Multiple international studies also corroborate the substantial direct costs for patients with AR, equivalent to approximately $200 per person per year in those countries[46,47]

Indirect costs are more difficult to accurately quantify. Among these costs is presenteeism, which is decreased productivity while present at work or school. There are several studies reporting the effects of AR on quality of life, especially as it results in sleep disturbance. Treatment of AR can reduce sleep disturbance, as determined by 2 systematic reviews and meta-analyses based on Epworth Sleepiness Score and Pittsburgh Sleep Quality Index.[48,49] AR has also been noted to contribute to at least $5 billion in lost productivity yearly,[50] with concern that presenteeism accounts for a fair amount of indirect cost.[51–53] Evidence also demonstrates its negative impact on mental health and school productivity[54–57] with a large meta-analysis concluding an odds ratio of 1.54 for patients with AR developing depression.[57] Overall, although difficult to quantify, AR appears to have substantial direct and indirect costs on the health care system.

SUMMARY

Asthma and AR are among the most commonly diagnosed and most prevalent medical conditions in the United States. Asthma and AR are often comorbid. AR is an independent risk factor for developing asthma. Up to 80% of people with asthma have AR, while asthma occurs in approximately 40% of people with AR. Diagnosis of asthma is more definitively obtained, and thus easier to study epidemiologically. On the other hand, the prevalence of AR is more difficult to accurately quantify as its symptom profile is more nonspecific and objective testing is less definitive. Multiple epidemiologic studies, however, demonstrate that the US prevalence of asthma is 8.7% among adults, and AR has a prevalence of at least 5% to 15% in the United States and 10% to 25% in Europe. Both account for significant, multi-billion-dollar health care burden which may continue to rise in the future.

CLINICS CARE POINTS

- The unified airway model suggests that inflammatory diseases of upper and lower airways are interconnected. AR affects up to 80% of people with asthma, and presence of asthma occurs in 40% of people with AR.
- Asthma is an obstructive pulmonary disorder with distinct symptoms of shortness of breath, cough, chest tightness, and/or wheezing.
- Asthma is a common diagnosis among adults and children, with prevalence of 8.7% among adults and 6.2% among children. Among adults and children with asthma, approximately 40% report at least 1 asthma exacerbation per year.
- Asthma accounts for significant health care costs in the United States, approximately $50 billion in medical costs and an additional $32 billion in indirect and mortality costs.
- AR is a heterogenous, IgE-mediated, type 1 hypersensitivity reaction in the nasal mucosa induced after allergen exposure to a sensitized individual. The IgE-mediated inflammatory response results in several symptoms, most commonly nasal congestion and rhinorrhea.
- Diagnosis of AR should rely on both history and objective testing, as testing in the absence of clinical history can lead to overdiagnosis and vice versa.
- Exact prevalence of AR is difficult to determine, but a combination of history and positive testing suggests a prevalence of between 5% and 15% in the United States.
- AR accounts for a significant health care cost burden, predominantly in terms of indirect costs related to reduced quality of life, as well as school and work productivity leading to presenteeism.

DISCLOSURE

The authors report no relevant financial disclosures.

REFERENCES

1. Seumois G, Zapardiel-Gonzalo J, White B, et al. Transcriptional Profiling of Th2 Cells Identifies Pathogenic Features Associated with Asthma. J Immunol 2016; 197(2):655–64.
2. Bachert C, Vignola AM, Gevaert P, et al. Allergic rhinitis, rhinosinusitis, and asthma: one airway disease. Immunol Allergy Clin North Am 2004;24(1):19–43.
3. Wise SK, Damask C, Roland LT, et al. International consensus statement on allergy and rhinology: Allergic rhinitis - 2023. Int Forum Allergy Rhinol 2023;13(4):293–859.
4. Corren J. Allergic rhinitis and asthma: how important is the link? J Allergy Clin Immunol. Feb 1997;99(2):S781–6.
5. Shen Y, Zeng JH, Hong SL, et al. Prevalence of allergic rhinitis comorbidity with asthma and asthma with allergic rhinitis in China: A meta-analysis. Asian Pac J Allergy Immunol 2019;37(4):220–5.
6. Pedersen CJ, Uddin MJ, Saha SK, et al. Prevalence of atopic dermatitis, asthma and rhinitis from infancy through adulthood in rural Bangladesh: a population-based, cross-sectional survey. BMJ Open 2020;10(11):e042380.
7. Tohidinik HR, Mallah N, Takkouche B. History of allergic rhinitis and risk of asthma; a systematic review and meta-analysis. World Allergy Organ J 2019;12(10):100069.
8. Ozoh OB, Aderibigbe SA, Ayuk AC, et al. The prevalence of asthma and allergic rhinitis in Nigeria: A nationwide survey among children, adolescents and adults. PLoS One 2019;14(9):e0222281.

9. Machluf Y, Farkash R, Rotkopf R, et al. Asthma phenotypes and associated co-morbidities in a large cohort of adolescents in Israel. J Asthma 2020;57(7): 722–35.
10. Testa D, M DIB, Nunziata M, et al. Allergic rhinitis and asthma assessment of risk factors in pediatric patients: A systematic review. Int J Pediatr Otorhinolaryngol 2020;129:109759.
11. Magnan A, Meunier JP, Saugnac C, et al. Frequency and impact of allergic rhinitis in asthma patients in everyday general medical practice: a French observational cross-sectional study. Allergy 2008;63(3):292–8.
12. de Groot EP, Nijkamp A, Duiverman EJ, et al. Allergic rhinitis is associated with poor asthma control in children with asthma. Thorax 2012;67(7):582–7.
13. Tay TR, Radhakrishna N, Hore-Lacy F, et al. Comorbidities in difficult asthma are independent risk factors for frequent exacerbations, poor control and diminished quality of life. Respirology 2016;21(8):1384–90.
14. Mims JW. Asthma: definitions and pathophysiology. Int Forum Allergy Rhinol 2015;5(Suppl 1):S2–6.
15. National Asthma E, Prevention P. Expert Panel Report 3 (EPR-3): Guidelines for the Diagnosis and Management of Asthma-Summary Report 2007. J Allergy Clin Immunol 2007;120(5 Suppl):S94–138.
16. Maslan J, Mims JW. What is asthma? Pathophysiology, demographics, and health care costs. Otolaryngol Clin North Am. 2014;47(1):13–22.
17. Corren J. Asthma phenotypes and endotypes: an evolving paradigm for classification. Discov Med 2013;15(83):243–9.
18. Cohn L, Elias JA, Chupp GL. Asthma: mechanisms of disease persistence and progression. Annu Rev Immunol 2004;22:789–815.
19. Handoyo S, Rosenwasser LJ. Asthma phenotypes. Curr Allergy Asthma Rep 2009;9(6):439–45.
20. Song P, Adeloye D, Salim H, et al. Global, regional, and national prevalence of asthma in 2019: a systematic analysis and modelling study. J Glob Health 2022;12:04052.
21. Nurmagambetov T, Kuwahara R, Garbe P. The Economic Burden of Asthma in the United States, 2008-2013. Ann Am Thorac Soc 2018;15(3):348–56.
22. Bousquet J, Khaltaev N, Cruz AA, et al. Allergic Rhinitis and its Impact on Asthma (ARIA) 2008 update (in collaboration with the World Health Organization, GA(2) LEN and AllerGen). Allergy 2008;63(Suppl 86):8–160.
23. Bousquet J, Schunemann HJ, Togias A, et al. Next-generation Allergic Rhinitis and Its Impact on Asthma (ARIA) guidelines for allergic rhinitis based on Grading of Recommendations Assessment, Development and Evaluation (GRADE) and real-world evidence. J Allergy Clin Immunol 2020;145(1):70–80 e3.
24. Bousquet J, Van Cauwenberge P, Khaltaev N, et al. Allergic rhinitis and its impact on asthma. J Allergy Clin Immunol 2001;108(5 Suppl):S147–334.
25. Mims JW. Epidemiology of allergic rhinitis. Int Forum Allergy Rhinol 2014;4(Suppl 2):S18–20.
26. Pastorello EA, Incorvaia C, Ortolani C, et al. Studies on the relationship between the level of specific IgE antibodies and the clinical expression of allergy: I. Definition of levels distinguishing patients with symptomatic from patients with asymptomatic allergy to common aeroallergens. J Allergy Clin Immunol 1995;96(5 Pt 1):580–7.
27. Graif Y, Goldberg A, Tamir R, et al. Skin test results and self-reported symptom severity in allergic rhinitis: The role of psychological factors. Clin Exp Allergy 2006;36(12):1532–7.

28. Oliveira TB, Persigo ALK, Ferrazza CC, et al. Prevalence of asthma, allergic rhinitis and pollinosis in a city of Brazil: A monitoring study. Allergol Immunopathol (Madr) 2020;48(6):537–44.

29. Alqahtani JM. Atopy and allergic diseases among Saudi young adults: A cross-sectional study. J Int Med Res. Jan 2020;48(1). https://doi.org/10.1177/03000605 19899760. 300060519899760.

30. Salo PM, Calatroni A, Gergen PJ, et al. Allergy-related outcomes in relation to serum IgE: results from the National Health and Nutrition Examination Survey 2005-2006. J Allergy Clin Immunol 2011;127(5):1226–12235 e7.

31. Tschopp JM, Sistek D, Schindler C, et al. Current allergic asthma and rhinitis: diagnostic efficiency of three commonly used atopic markers (IgE, skin prick tests, and Phadiatop). Results from 8329 randomized adults from the SAPALDIA Study. Swiss Study on Air Pollution and Lung Diseases in Adults. Allergy 1998; 53(6):608–13.

32. Arbes SJ Jr, Gergen PJ, Elliott L, et al. Prevalences of positive skin test responses to 10 common allergens in the US population: results from the third National Health and Nutrition Examination Survey. J Allergy Clin Immunol 2005;116(2): 377–83.

33. Nam JS, Hwang CS, Hong MP, et al. Prevalence and clinical characteristics of allergic rhinitis in the elderly Korean population. Eur Arch Oto-Rhino-Laryngol 2020;277(12):3367–73.

34. Mortz CG, Andersen KE, Poulsen LK, et al. Atopic diseases and type I sensitization from adolescence to adulthood in an unselected population (TOACS) with focus on predictors for allergic rhinitis. Allergy 2019;74(2):308–17.

35. Wang XY, Ma TT, Wang XY, et al. Prevalence of pollen-induced allergic rhinitis with high pollen exposure in grasslands of northern China. Allergy 2018;73(6): 1232–43.

36. Ait-Khaled N, Pearce N, Anderson HR, et al. Global map of the prevalence of symptoms of rhinoconjunctivitis in children: The International Study of Asthma and Allergies in Childhood (ISAAC) Phase Three. Allergy 2009;64(1):123–48.

37. Bjorksten B, Clayton T, Ellwood P, et al. Worldwide time trends for symptoms of rhinitis and conjunctivitis: Phase III of the International Study of Asthma and Allergies in Childhood. Pediatr Allergy Immunol 2008;19(2):110–24.

38. Strachan D, Sibbald B, Weiland S, et al. Worldwide variations in prevalence of symptoms of allergic rhinoconjunctivitis in children: the International Study of Asthma and Allergies in Childhood (ISAAC). Pediatr Allergy Immunol 1997;8(4): 161–76.

39. Weinmayr G, Forastiere F, Weiland SK, et al. International variation in prevalence of rhinitis and its relationship with sensitisation to perennial and seasonal allergens. Eur Respir J 2008;32(5):1250–61.

40. Ronmark E, Bjerg A, Perzanowski M, et al. Major increase in allergic sensitization in schoolchildren from 1996 to 2006 in northern Sweden. J Allergy Clin Immunol 2009;124(2):357–63, 63 e1-15.

41. Goetzel RZ, Long SR, Ozminkowski RJ, et al. Health, absence, disability, and presenteeism cost estimates of certain physical and mental health conditions affecting U.S. employers. J Occup Environ Med 2004;46(4):398–412.

42. Meltzer EO, Bukstein DA. The economic impact of allergic rhinitis and current guidelines for treatment. Ann Allergy Asthma Immunol 2011;106(2 Suppl):S12–6.

43. Roland LT, Wise SK, Wang H, et al. The cost of rhinitis in the United States: a national insurance claims analysis. Int Forum Allergy Rhinol 2021;11(5):946–8.

44. Workman AD, Dattilo L, Rathi VK, et al. Contemporary Incremental Healthcare Costs for Allergic Rhinitis in the United States. Laryngoscope 2022;132(8):1510–4.
45. Law AW, Reed SD, Sundy JS, et al. Direct costs of allergic rhinitis in the United States: estimates from the 1996 Medical Expenditure Panel Survey. J Allergy Clin Immunol 2003;111(2):296–300.
46. Avdeeva KS, Reitsma S, Fokkens WJ. Direct and indirect costs of allergic and non-allergic rhinitis in the Netherlands. Allergy 2020;75(11):2993–6.
47. Cardell LO, Olsson P, Andersson M, et al. TOTALL: high cost of allergic rhinitis-a national Swedish population-based questionnaire study. NPJ Prim Care Respir Med 2016;26:15082.
48. Liu J, Zhang X, Zhao Y, et al. The association between allergic rhinitis and sleep: A systematic review and meta-analysis of observational studies. PLoS One 2020; 15(2):e0228533.
49. Fried J, Yuen E, Zhang K, et al. Impact of Treatment for Nasal Cavity Disorders on Sleep Quality: Systematic Review and Meta-analysis. Otolaryngol Head Neck Surg 2022;166(4):633–42.
50. Crystal-Peters J, Crown WH, Goetzel RZ, et al. The cost of productivity losses associated with allergic rhinitis. Am J Manag Care 2000;6(3):373–8.
51. Colas C, Brosa M, Anton E, et al. Estimate of the total costs of allergic rhinitis in specialized care based on real-world data: the FERIN Study. Allergy 2017;72(6): 959–66.
52. Vandenplas O, Vinnikov D, Blanc PD, et al. Impact of Rhinitis on Work Productivity: A Systematic Review. J Allergy Clin Immunol Pract 2018;6(4):1274–1286 e9.
53. Lamb CE, Ratner PH, Johnson CE, et al. Economic impact of workplace productivity losses due to allergic rhinitis compared with select medical conditions in the United States from an employer perspective. Curr Med Res Opin 2006;22(6): 1203–10.
54. Hoehle LP, Speth MM, Phillips KM, et al. Association between symptoms of allergic rhinitis with decreased general health-related quality of life. Am J Rhinol Allergy 2017;31(4):235–9.
55. Mir E, Panjabi C, Shah A. Impact of allergic rhinitis in school going children. Asia Pac Allergy 2012;2(2):93–100.
56. Trikojat K, Buske-Kirschbaum A, Plessow F, et al. Memory and multitasking performance during acute allergic inflammation in seasonal allergic rhinitis. Clin Exp Allergy 2017;47(4):479–87.
57. Wang J, Xiao D, Chen H, et al. Cumulative evidence for association of rhinitis and depression. Allergy Asthma Clin Immunol 2021;17(1):111.

Incorporating Asthma Evaluation into the Otolaryngic Allergy Practice
Presentation and Diagnosis

Cecelia Damask, DO[a], Christine Franzese, MD[b],*

KEYWORDS

- Asthma • Allergic rhinitis • Asthma phenotypes • Spirometry • FeNO

KEY POINTS

- Eliciting a history of wheezing, shortness of breath, chest tightness, and coughing is a vital part of the presentation of asthma, which can present with different phenotypes.
- Symptoms may vary over time and physical examination may not always elicit findings so further diagnostic evaluation is important.
- Pulmonary function testing, spirometry, fractional exhaled nitric oxide, and impulse oscillometry can aid in objective measurements and the correct diagnosis of asthma.

INTRODUCTION

In any allergy practice, patients presenting for atopic symptoms will frequently have one or more associated comorbid condition[s]. Among those, asthma is one of the most common, with up to 38% of patients with allergic rhinitis having asthma as well.[1] However, not all patients with symptoms suspicious for asthma will carry the official diagnosis. Because asthma occurs in all age ranges and its prevalence seems to be increasing globally, it is highly likely that a practicing otolaryngologist will see a considerable number of patients with asthma regardless of whether the practice includes allergic diseases or not.[1]

The understanding of asthma has evolved during the decades from a disorder of not only bronchoconstriction but also one driven by chronic inflammation of the lower airways involving tissue remodeling and airway hyperresponsiveness.[2] As the understanding of asthma improves, awareness has also evolved to recognize that asthma

[a] Department of Otolaryngology, Orlando ENT & Allergy, University of Central Florida, 11317 Lake Underhill Road, Suite 100, Orlando, FL 32825, USA; [b] Department of Otolaryngology-Head and Neck Surgery, University of Missouri-Columbia, One Hospital Drive, Suite MA314, Columbia, MO 65212, USA
* Corresponding author.
E-mail address: franzesec@umsystem.edu

Otolaryngol Clin N Am 57 (2024) 191–199
https://doi.org/10.1016/j.otc.2023.09.002
0030-6665/24/© 2023 Elsevier Inc. All rights reserved.

is a heterogeneous disease process that can be driven by different underlying pathologic conditions.[3] This variability can make the diagnosis and treatment of asthma challenging. Although evaluating patients for and making the diagnosis of asthma may seem extraneous to an otolaryngology practice, it can be extremely beneficial to patients and have important repercussions for the allergy portion of the practice itself.

Even if a decision is made by the provider not to participate in asthma management, the ability to recognize the various presentations of asthma, diagnose it, and assess a patient's asthma severity and control is still extremely important. Poorly controlled or uncontrolled asthma increases the risk of having an adverse event for those patients receiving subcutaneous immunotherapy. Exacerbations or increased symptoms occurring outside of immunotherapy injections can contribute to potential delays in escalation or failure to achieve maintenance dosing due to the patient missing one or more injections when symptoms worsen.

PRESENTATION

Clinical history taking remains a vital part of diagnosing asthma but can prove challenging for several reasons. Just as our understanding of asthma has evolved, so too has the recognition that there may be variability in clinical presentations due to different phenotypes/endotypes. Asthma can present in younger and in older patients, in those with a history of allergies and in those without, as well as in those with conditions such as obesity. Adding to the challenge is the fact that those with symptoms of asthma tend to underreport those symptoms to their providers, contributing to the underdiagnosis of asthma. Recent population-based studies of adults and children suggest that 7% to 10% of the adult and pediatric populations have current asthma, and in those with current asthma, 20% to 73% remain undiagnosed.[4] Specifically asking questions to elicit respiratory symptoms and then evaluating with objective diagnostic testing may help reduce the underdiagnosis of asthma.[4]

According to the Global Initiative in Asthma, asthma is defined by a history of respiratory symptoms such as wheeze, shortness of breath, chest tightness, and cough that vary over time and in intensity, together with variable airflow limitation.[3] These symptoms, airflow restriction, and activity restriction may be quiescent for extended periods and then may suddenly occur with a trigger, or may worsen as an exacerbation of chronically mild symptoms, or anywhere in between. Common triggers for asthmatics can include viral respiratory illnesses, physical activity/exercise, and smoke or allergen exposure, among others.

Although this definition may seem relatively simple and straightforward, asthma is now considered an umbrella diagnosis encompassing different underlying inflammatory pathophysiologies, which can be expressed in various diverse phenotypes.[4] What is considered an asthma "phenotype" has evolved over time as well. Initial perceptions of phenotypes were related to allergy/atopic status, with asthma being either extrinsic/allergic or intrinsic/nonallergic phenotype.[5] Over time, this perception has evolved to one that groups phenotypes related to or driven by a mechanistic disease process, such as aspirin exacerbated respiratory disease.[6] Currently, there is some controversy over how many different asthma phenotypes exist but, in essence, the most widely recognized phenotypes are based on the type of inflammation, age of onset, and associated conditions such as obesity and elevated eosinophils.[6]

Several multicenter studies[7–9] using different clustering techniques to identify asthma phenotypes in large cohorts have identified approximately 4 primary asthma phenotypes.[10] Although significant differences exist in the cohorts evaluated, disease features assessed, and the statistical approaches used in each study, the studies' results seem to suggest the 4 phenotypes: early-onset mild allergic asthma, early-onset allergic moderate-to-severe remodeled asthma, late-onset nonallergic eosinophilic asthma, and late-onset noneosinophilic nonallergic asthma.[7-10]

Early onset allergic phenotypes are considered to be the most common asthma phenotypes in the pediatric population.[5] The early-onset mild phenotype typically presents with intermittent or less-severe symptoms, whereas the early-onset allergic moderate-to-severe remodeled phenotype can present from mild to severe.[5] There is no definitive age associated with either "early-onset"" phenotype. It is unclear if the early-onset mild allergic phenotype continues or evolves into adulthood.[5] It is also unknown if the early-onset allergic moderate-to-severe remodeled phenotype progresses from a milder form or instead originates de novo during childhood.[11] Both of these phenotypes are distinguished by positive allergy skin tests and increased serum-specific immunoglobulin (Ig) E. The mild form demonstrates preservation of lung function on spirometry, whereas the moderate-to-severe remodeled form demonstrates reduced lung function.[5,11]

Similar to the early-onset phenotypes, there is no specific age associated with the late-onset phenotypes other than that they occur in adults. Unlike the early-onset phenotypes, the later-onset phenotypes tend to have a more severe presentation and have an association with female sex and obesity.[10] The eosinophilic phenotypes demonstrate Type 2 (T2) airway inflammation that is driven by a variety of cytokines, including interleukins 4, 5, and 13, and features elevated eosinophils and IgE, among other biomakers.[12] The noneosinophilic phenotypes involve low T2/non-T2 inflammatory cascades that feature more neutrophilic inflammation. A subset of late-onset nonallergic eosinophilic asthmatics has a distinct steroid-resistant eosinophilic phenotype of unknown molecular mechanism, which tends to present with more severe asthma with fixed airflow obstruction.[13] This phenotype (late-onset nonallergic eosinophilic) has the strongest association with comorbid chronic sinusitis with nasal polyps (CRSwNP). In patients with CRSwNP and late-onset nonallergic eosinophilic asthma, the nasal polyps will typically present before the development of asthma.[5]

Regardless of whether a patient conforms to a specific phenotype, if respiratory symptoms suspicious for asthma are elicited during the patient history, further diagnostic testing should be pursued.

DIAGNOSIS

Asthma continues to be a diagnostic challenge because its clinical signs and symptoms are nonspecific and can be difficult to distinguish from other respiratory conditions. A key diagnostic feature of asthma is that symptom severity varies over time. It is important for the otolaryngologist to ask about the patient's symptoms as well as the timing of those symptoms. Characteristically, the symptoms of asthma are intermittent; they can vary throughout the day with worsening often seen in the evening and early morning. Symptoms may also vary seasonally. There are specific triggers that have been associated with asthma including pollen, animal dander, cold temperature, exercise, aspirin and nonsteroidal anti-inflammatory drugs, and certain occupational exposures.

A carefully elicited history is paramount in the diagnosis of asthma because the physical examination may not offer many clues due to the episodic nature of asthma. The otolaryngologist should listen for wheezing on auscultation both during tidal respiration as well as during forced expiration. Care should also be taken to determine if the expiratory phase of breathing is prolonged.

Spirometry

Spirometry is a physiologic test measuring the volume of air that an individual can inspire and expire with maximal effort. The primary parameter measured in spirometry is either volume or flow as a function of time. The most relevant measurements include the forced vital capacity (FVC), which is the volume delivered during an expiration made as forcefully and completely as possible starting from full inspiration, and the forced expiratory volume (FEV1), which is the expiratory volume in the first second of an FVC maneuver.[14] Spirometry is valuable as a screening test of general respiratory health much like blood pressure provides valuable information about general cardiovascular health. However, spirometry alone does not lead directly to a diagnosis of asthma.

Performing spirometry can be physically demanding with the forced expiratory maneuver resulting in increased intrathoracic, intra-abdominal, and intracranial pressures.[15,16] As a result, there are some relative contraindications to spirometry requiring caution in patients with medical conditions that could be adversely affected by pressures generated in the thorax. Patients also should avoid certain activities before spirometry, and they should be informed of these activities before the test. **Boxes 1** and **2** review relative contraindications for spirometry and activities that should be avoided before lung function testing, respectively.

Before performing spirometry, the patient's age and height are recorded. Their height should be measured without shoes, standing as tall as possible. Birth sex and ethnicity should be recorded. Although gender identity should be respected, it is believed that the use of biological sex will yield a more accurate prediction of lung function because the effect of gender-affirming hormonal therapy on lung function is poorly understood.[17] Assigning ethnicity is challenging. Ethnicity categories for the Global Lung Function Initiative (GLI) reference values[18] are White (ie, European ancestry), African American, Northeast Asian, Southeast Asian, and other/mixed **(Table 1)**. The differences by population groupings that were observed in the GLI data could represent genetic differences but potentially may just highlight underlying health disparities. Therefore, the specific contribution that genetic ancestry plays in the regional differences that were observed in GLI data remains unclear.

The patient should be given a nose clip to wear and make sure that their lips are sealed around the mouthpiece. During spirometry, a patient inspires maximally to total lung capacity (TLC), and then exhales forcefully, rapidly, and as completely as possible into spirometer. There are 4 distinct phases of the FVC maneuver: (1) maximal inspiration, (2) a "blast" of expiration, (3) continued complete expiration for a maximum of 15 seconds, and (4) inspiration at maximal flow back to maximum lung volume on spirometers that measure inspiration and expiration. Most of the variability in results obtained from spirometry relates to inadequate and variable inspiration to TLC, ending the expiration prematurely, and variable effort. At full inflation, without hesitation, the patient should then be prompted to "blast," not just "blow," all the air from their lungs. Continuous and enthusiastic coaching of the patient is required throughout the maneuver.

Bronchodilator responsiveness (BDR) testing is a determination of the degree of improvement of airflow in response to bronchodilator administration as measured by changes in FEV1 and FVC. It is commonly undertaken as part of spirometry testing. A bronchodilator is administered and after a wait time, 3 or more additional postbronchodilator FEV1 and FVC measurements are then obtained. Changes in FEV1 and FVC following BDR testing are expressed as the percent change relative to the individual's predicted value. A change greater than 10% of the predicted value indicates a positive response.[17]

Box 1
Relative Contraindications for Spirometry

Due to increases in myocardial demand or changes in blood pressure
  Acute myocardial infarction within 1 wk
  Systemic hypotension or severe hypertension
  Significant atria/ventricular arrhythmia
  Noncompensated heart failure
  Uncontrolled pulmonary hypertension
  Acute cor pulmonale
  Clinically unstable pulmonary embolism
  History of syncope related to forced expiration/cough

Due to increases in intracranial/intraocular pressure
  Cerebral aneurysm
  Brain surgery within 4 wk
  Recent concussion with continuing symptoms
  Eye surgery within 1 wk

Due to increases in sinus and middle ear pressures
  Sinus surgery or middle ear surgery or infection within 1 wk

Due to increases in intrathoracic and intra-abdominal pressure
  Presence of pneumothorax
  Thoracic surgery within 4 wk
  Abdominal surgery within 4 wk
  Late-term pregnancy

Infection control issues
  Active or suspected transmissible respiratory or systemic infection, including tuberculosis

Physical conditions predisposing to transmission of infections, such as hemoptysis, significant secretions, or oral lesions or oral bleeding

Spirometry should be discontinued if the patient experiences pain during the maneuver. Relative contraindications do not preclude spirometry but should be considered when ordering spirometry. The decision to conduct spirometry is determined by the ordering health-care professional because of their evaluation of the risks and benefits of spirometry for the particular patient. Potential contraindications should be included in the request form for spirometry.

The largest FVC and the largest FEV1 observed from all of the acceptable values are reported. Their ratio is used for FEV1/FVC, even though the largest FVC and the largest FEV1 may not necessarily come from the same maneuver. If a bronchodilator is administered, both the percentage change and the absolute change in FEV1 and FVC compared with prebronchodilator values are reported.[19]

The ERS/ATS technical standard on interpretive strategies for routine lung function tests states that the interpretation of technically acceptable pulmonary function test results has 3 key aspects, which are distinct yet complementary.[17]

1. Classification of observed values as within/outside the normal range with respect to a population of healthy individuals, considering the measurement error of the test, as well as the inherent biological variability of measurements both between individuals and between repeated measurements in the same individual.

Box 2
Activities That Should Be Avoided Before Lung Function Testing

- Smoking and/or vaping and/or water pipe use within 1 h before testing (to avoid acute bronchoconstriction due to smoke inhalation)
- Consuming intoxicants within 8 h before testing (to avoid problems in coordination, comprehension, and physical ability)
- Performing vigorous exercise within 1 h before testing (to avoid potential exercise-induced bronchoconstriction)
- Wearing clothing that substantially restricts full chest and abdominal expansion (to avoid external restrictions on lung function)

Reprinted with permission of the American Thoracic Society. Copyright © 2023 American Thoracic Society. All rights reserved. Graham BL, et al. Standardization of Spirometry 2019 Update. An Official American Thoracic Society and European Respiratory Society Technical Statement. Am J Respir Crit Care Med. 2019 Oct 15;200(8):e70-e88. The American Journal of Respiratory and Critical Care Medicine is an official journal of the American Thoracic Society.

---

2. Integration of knowledge of physiologic determinants of test results into a functional classification of the identified impairments.
3. Integration of the identified patterns with other clinical data to inform differential diagnosis and guide therapy.

A reference range represents the distribution of values that are expected in a healthy population and the lower limit of normal (LLN) represents a cut-off to define results that are outside the range of values typically observed in health.[17] With spirometry, it has become standard to define the LLN as the fifth percentile. The LLN provides an indication of whether the observed result can be expected in otherwise healthy individuals of similar age, sex, and height.

Airflow limitation and airflow obstruction can be assessed by spirometry with important indices being FVC, FEV1, and the FEV1/FVC ratio. The FEV1/FVC ratio helps to determine whether an obstruction is present or not; an obstructive ventilatory impairment is defined by FEV1/FVC below the LLN.[17] If the FEV1/FVC ratio is normal, then we look at the FVC. If the FVC is normal, then the spirometry is interpreted as normal, whereas if the FVC is less than the LLN, then there may be restriction present.

Fractional Exhaled Nitric Oxide

Measurement of fractional exhaled nitric oxide (FeNO) is a noninvasive technique used to determine eosinophilic airway inflammation and can be used as a tool to assist with the diagnosis and management of asthma. Nitric oxide (NO) is produced by respiratory epithelial cells, with NO production increased in response to inflammatory cytokines in the airways.[20] NO is present in exhaled breath, and measurements have been demonstrated to correlate with sputum eosinophil level.[21] FeNO can be easily measured in children and has potential to be useful in the diagnosis and management of asthma in children, especially those too young to perform spirometry.[22]

Impulse Oscillometry

Another tool that may be helpful in providing objective information in children diagnosed with or suspected to have asthma is impulse oscillometry (IOS). Children aged younger than 5 years are rarely able to perform a skilled test such as spirometry

Table 1
Summary of global lung function initiative equations for spirometry and current evidence regarding application of these equations in different populations

GLI reference population	GLI data source	Population/ ancestral origin	Considerations
White	Europe, Israel, Australia, USA, Canada, Brazil, Chile, Mexico, Uruguay, Venezuela, Algeria, and Tunisia	White (European) Hispanic (European)	Suitable for use in White European populations [36,175,176]
Black	African American	Black (North America)	
South East Asian	Thailand, Taiwan, and China (including Hong Kong)	Asian	
North East Asian	Japan and Korea		North East Asian equations demonstrate poor fit when applied to contemporary populations [29]
Multiethnic	Average of the other 4 GLI groups	Multiracial, Black, South Africa [177]; India [178]; unknown	India [178] and South African [177] data based on a single prospective study in children

From: Stanojevic S, Kaminsky DA, Miller MR, Thompson B, Aliverti A, Barjaktarevic I, Cooper BG, Culver B, Derom E, Hall GL, Hallstrand TS, Leuppi JD, MacIntyre N, McCormack M, Rosenfeld M, Swenson ER. ERS/ATS technical standard on interpretive strategies for routine lung function tests. Eur Respir J. 2022 Jul 13;60(1):2101499. https://doi.org/10.1183/13993003.01499-2021. PMID: 34949706.

resulting in preschool asthma most often diagnosed and managed based on clinical findings. IOS is a lung function test that can be performed by younger children and those unable to perform spirometry. IOS requires minimal cooperation with measurements made during tidal breathing. IOS uses sound waves to transmit pressure into the airways and thereby determine pressure and flow over a range of frequencies.

Table 2
Objective testing methods aiding in asthma diagnosis

Objective Test Method	What is Measured	How These Aid in Diagnosis
Spirometry	Measures either volume or flow as a function of time	Allow for calculation of airflow limitation and airflow obstruction
FeNO	Measures NO in exhaled breath	Determines eosinophilic airway inflammation
IOS	Determines pressure and flow over a range of frequency	Allow objective calculations in patients unable to perform skilled tests such as spirometry (ie, children <5 y)

Once pressure and flow have been determined, other characteristics of the airway, such as resistance, can be calculated.[22]

There are several objective testing methods that can aid in asthma diagnosis. **Table 2** compares these various methods.

SUMMARY

Recognizing the presentation of asthma, its various phenotypes, and associated comorbidities serves as an important part of any allergy practice. Diagnosing asthma and understanding its ramifications can benefit both patients and providers. The heterogeneous inflammatory processes that drive the symptoms of asthma result in a variety of phenotypic presentations. Recognizing the most common phenotypic forms can facilitate obtaining objective diagnostic testing. Diagnostic testing, including spirometry and other objective respiratory tests, is integral to not only making the diagnosis of asthma but also improving the accuracy of its diagnosis.

CLINICS CARE POINTS

- Taking the time to elicit a history of respiratory symptoms, such as wheezing, shortness of breath, chest tightness, and cough that vary over time and in intensity is an important step in making the diagnosis of asthma.
- Auscultation for wheezing is an important component of the physician examination but because wheezing may not always be present, follow up with objective measurements.
- Objective measurement of airflow limitation and airflow obstruction can be assessed by spirometry with important indices being FVC, FEV1, and the FEV1/FVC ratio.

DISCLOSURE

C. Damask: Advisory Board-Genentech, Grifols, GSK, Sanofi/Regeneron; Clinical Research-AstraZeneca, GSK, OptiNose, Regeneron; Speakers Bureau-AstraZeneca, GSK, OptiNose, Sanofi/Regeneron. C. Franzese: Speakers Bureau-GSK, AZ, Optinose, Regeneron, Sanofi; Advisory Board-Sanofi; Research Funding-GSK, AZ, Optinose, Regeneron, United States, Sanofi, United States, Biohaven, Bellus, Lyra.

REFERENCES

1. Brożek JL, Bousquet J, Agache L, et al. Allergic rhinitis and its impact on asthma (ARIA) guidelines-2016 revision. J. Allergy Clin. Immunol 2017;140(4):950–8.
2. Franzese C, Damask CC, Franzese C, et al. SK. Handbook of otolaryngic allergy. New York: Thieme; 2019. p. 194–9.
3. Global Initiative for Asthma. Global Strategy for Asthma Management and Prevention, 2023. 2023. Available at: www.ginasthma.org.
4. Aaron SD, Boulet LP, Reddel HK, et al. Underdiagnosis and overdiagnosis of asthma. Am J Respir Crit Care Med 2018;198(8):1012–20.
5. Kuruvilla ME, Lee FE, Lee GB. Understanding asthma phenotypes, endotypes, and mechanisms of disease. Clin Rev Allergy Immunol 2019;56(2):219–33.
6. Wenzel S. Asthma phenotypes: the evolution from clinical to molecular approaches. Nat Med 2012;18:716–25.
7. Moore WC, Meyers DA, Wenzel SE, et al. Identification of asthma phenotypes using cluster analysis in the Severe Asthma Research Program. Am J Respir Crit Care Med 2010;181:315–23.

8. Haldar P, Pavord ID, Shaw DE, et al. Cluster analysis and clinical asthma pheno-types. Am J Respir Crit Care Med 2008;178:218–24.
9. Lefaudeux D, De Meulder B, Loza MJ, et al. U-BIOPRED clinical adult asthma clusters linked to a subset of sputum omics. J Allergy Clin Immunol 2017;139: 1797–807.
10. Kaur R, Chupp G. Phenotypes and endotypes of adult asthma: Moving toward precision medicine. J Allergy Clin Immunol 2019;144(1):1–12.
11. Miranda C, Busacker A, Balzar S, et al. Distinguishing severe asthma pheno-types: role of age at onset and eosinophilic inflammation. J Allergy Clin Immunol 2004;113(1):101–8.
12. Dunican EM, Fahy JV. The role of type 2 inflammation in the pathogenesis of asthma exacerbations. Ann Am Thorac Soc. 2015;12(Suppl 2):S144–9.
13. Peters MC, Kerr S, Dunican EM, et al. National heart, lung and blood institute se-vere asthma research program 3. Refractory airway type 2 inflammation in a large subgroup of asthmatic patients treated with inhaled corticosteroids. J Allergy Clin Immunol 2019;143(1):104–13.
14. Miller MR, Hankinson J, Brusasco V, et al. ATS/ERS task force. standardisation of spirometry. Eur Respir J 2005;26(2):319–38.
15. Cooper BG. An update on contraindications for lung function testing. Thorax 2011;66:714–23.
16. Tiller NB, Simpson AJ. Effect of spirometry on intra-thoracic pressures. BMC Res Notes 2018;11:110.
17. Stanojevic S, Kaminsky DA, Miller MR, et al. ERS/ATS technical standard on inter-pretive strategies for routine lung function tests. Eur Respir J 2022;60(1): 2101499.
18. Quanjer PH, Stanojevic S, Cole TJ, et al. ERS global lung function initiative. multi-ethnic reference values for spirometry for the 3–95-yr age range: the global lung function 2012 equations. Eur Respir J 2012;40:1324–43.
19. Graham BL, Steenbruggen I, Miller MR, et al. Standardization of spirometry 2019 update. an official american thoracic society and european respiratory society technical statement. Am J Respir Crit Care Med 2019;200(8):e70–88.
20. Moncada S, Higgs A. The L-arginine nitric oxide pathway. N Engl J Med 1993; 329:2002–12.
21. Payne DN, Adcock IM, Wilson NM, et al. Relationship between exhaled nitric ox-ide and mucosal eosinophilic inflammation in children with difficult asthma after treatment with oral prednisolone. Am J Respir Crit Care Med 2001;164:1376–81.
22. McDowell KM. Recent diagnosis techniques in pediatric asthma: impulse oscill-ometry in preschool asthma and use of exhaled nitric oxide. Immunol Allergy Clin North Am. 2019;39(2):205–19.

Interpretation of Spirometry, Peak Flow, and Provocation Testing for Asthma

Sukhmani Boparai, MBBS, MD[a], George M. Solomon, MD[a,b,c,d],*

KEYWORDS

- Asthma • Spirometry • Bronchodilator testing • Bronchoprovocation testing
- Fractional exhaled nitric oxide • Peak flow

KEY POINTS

- Asthma diagnosis depends on recognizing respiratory symptoms and demonstrating variable expiratory airflow limitation through spirometry. Various methods, including peak flow and bronchodilator and bronchoprovocation testing, are used to exhibit this variability.
- A positive bronchodilator response is diagnostic of asthma within the appropriate clinical context.
- Bronchoprovocation testing aids in diagnosing asthma by revealing smooth muscle hyperactivity when spirometry results are inconclusive.
- Fractional exhaled nitric oxide and peak flow can serve as adjuncts for asthma diagnosis but have several limitations.
- Asthma diagnosis presents numerous challenges, underscoring the importance of early testing and a multifaceted diagnostic approach.

DEFINING ASTHMA

Diagnosis of asthma is based on identifying a typical/characteristic pattern of respiratory symptoms such as wheezing, shortness of breath/dyspnea, chest tightness or cough, and variable expiratory airflow limitation (**Fig. 1**). Spirometry is essential for demonstrating and documenting evidence of excessive variability in lung function and expiratory airflow limitation.

[a] UAB Division of Pulmonary, Allergy, and Critical Care Medicine, University of Alabama at Birmingham, Pulmonary and Critical Care Medicine, 1900 University Boulevard, THT 422, Birmingham, AL 35294, USA; [b] UAB Adult PCD and Bronchiectasis Programs; [c] UAB CF Therapeutics Development Network Center; [d] Gregory Fleming James CF Research Center, Birmingham, AL, USA
* Corresponding author. Gregory Fleming James CF Research Center, Birmingham, AL.
E-mail address: gsolomon@uabmc.edu

Otolaryngol Clin N Am 57 (2024) 201–213
https://doi.org/10.1016/j.otc.2023.12.001
0030-6665/24/© 2023 Elsevier Inc. All rights reserved.

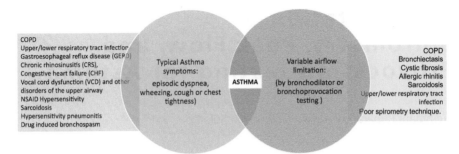

Fig. 1. Overlap of clinical features and spirometry required for diagnosis of asthma.

It is crucial to obtain spirometry early to avoid misdiagnosis with other serious cardiopulmonary diseases and to avoid underdiagnosis or overdiagnosis and treatment.[1]

BASIC CONCEPTS IN SPIROMETRY/PULMONARY FUNCTION TESTING

Pulmonary function tests (PFTs) reflect the physiologic properties of the lungs (eg, airflow mechanics, volumes, and gas transfer). They are used to diagnose lung disease, explain dyspnea, and monitor disease progression and treatment response.

Spirometry is a component of PFTs that estimates the volume of air inhaled or exhaled using a pneumotachometer to measure flow rates during ventilatory maneuvers.

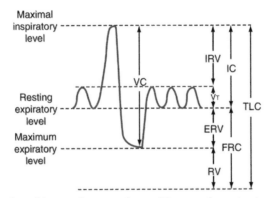

Fig. 2. Representation of lung volumes and capacities on spirometry. Lung volume and capacity. There are four volumes, which do not overlap[1]: tidal volume (Vt) is the volume of gas inhaled or exhaled during each respiratory cycle[2]; inspiratory reserve volume (IRV) is the maximal volume of gas inspired from end inspiration[3]; expiratory reserve volume (ERV) is the maximal volume of gas exhaled from end expiration; and[4] residual volume (RV) is the volume of gas remaining in the lungs after a maximal exhalation. There are four capacities, each of which contains two or more primary volumes[1]: total lung capacity (TLC) is the amount of gas contained in the lung at maximal inspiration[2]; vital capacity (VC) is the maximal volume of gas that can be expelled from the lungs after maximal inspiration, without regard for the time involved[3]; inspiratory capacity (IC) is the maximal volume of gas that can be inspired from the resting expiratory level; and[4] functional residual capacity (FRC) is the volume of gas in the lungs at resting end expiration. (*From* Broaddus VC, Ernst JD, King TE, et al. Murray & Nadel's Textbook of Respiratory Medicine. 7 ed. vol 1. Elsevier; 2022.)

Maneuvers performed using maximal expiratory effort are called forced maneuvers. Lung volumes and capacities are defined as shown in **Fig. 2**.

It is essential to understand that PFTs do not diagnose specific diseases. Instead, the different patterns of abnormalities seen in PFTs can classify pulmonary dysfunction into categories such as obstructive, restrictive, mixed, or nonspecific ventilatory defects and guide further evaluation. The testing equipment and maneuvers should meet the recommended protocols and criteria for acceptability. Another caveat to interpreting PFTs is that many maneuvers depend on patient effort and understanding.[2]

SPIROMETRY IN ASTHMA

In asthma, spirometry may be normal or show airflow obstruction, especially when a patient is symptomatic.

Airflow obstruction is defined by a decrease in forced expiratory volume in one second (FEV1)/forced vital capacity (FVC) less than 0.70 or less than lower limits or normal with a reduced FEV1 and a normal (or reduced) FVC. The expiratory flow–volume curve shows a characteristic upward concavity (**Fig. 3**)

However, the more characteristic spirometry finding of asthma is the expiratory airflow variability, that is, improvement and/or deterioration in symptoms and lung function. This is more pronounced asthma as compared with healthy individuals. Excessive variability may be identified more than 1 day (diurnal variability), from day to day, from visit to visit, seasonally, from a reversibility test, or after initiating treatment with bronchodilators.

Objectively demonstrating airway variability is the cornerstone of asthma diagnosis and can be done in multiple ways: peak flow, bronchodilator response, or bronchoprovocation testing, as discussed later in this article.[2]

Some other caveats to remember while interpreting spirometry for diagnosing asthma are.

1. There is a broad differential for airway obstruction on spirometry, including chronic obstructive pulmonary disease (COPD), bronchiectasis, cystic fibrosis, bronchitis, or poor spirometry technique.
2. As in COPD, using a fixed cutoff of FEV1/FVC less than 0.70 to define obstruction may misclassify patients due to differences in demographics or other factors

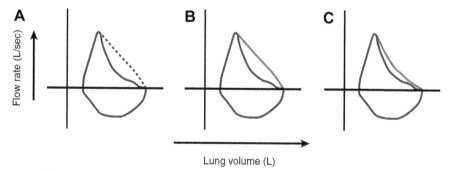

Fig. 3. Flow volume loops in asthma: Solid blue line shows the typical scooped appearance in asthma. (*A*) Dashed blue line shows predicted normal flow volume, (*B*) yellow line shows complete reversal following bronchodilator, and (*C*) yellow line shows incomplete reversal following bronchodilator. (*From* Mathur SK, Busse WW. Asthma: diagnosis and management. Med Clin North Am. 2006;90(1):39-60. * Elsevier.)

3. Airflow obstruction and variability may be masked if bronchodilator treatment is started before testing, thus confounding the diagnosis.

In the following sections, the authors discuss tests used to demonstrate expiratory airflow variability and hyperresponsiveness.

BRONCHODILATOR TESTING

Bronchodilator testing is used to assess changes in expiratory airflow in response to an inhaled bronchodilator. In the appropriate clinical context, a positive response is suggestive of a diagnosis of asthma. This test involves performing baseline spirometry followed by an inhaled bronchodilator—commonly albuterol (180 µg) and then repeating spirometry after 10 to 20 minutes.

According to the 2019/2022 American Thoracic Society/European Respiratory Society (ATS/ERS) statement, a change in post-bronchodilator FEV1 and FVC greater than 10% of the predicted value is considered a positive test (**Box 1**).

This was a change from the 2005 ATS/ERS guidelines, which defined a positive response as a combination of an absolute and relative change (percentage change) in FEV1 and FVC from baseline as evidence of bronchodilator response (BDR) (ie, >200 mL AND $\not\leq$12% increase in FEV1 and/or FVC). This change incorporated evidence suggesting that the absolute and relative changes in FEV1 and FVC are inversely proportional to baseline lung function and are associated with height, age, and sex. This approach avoids misinterpretation due to the magnitude of the baseline lung function level.[3]

BDR differs from the "reversibility" of airflow obstruction, which refers to the normalization of FEV1/FVC after bronchodilator administration.

Other considerations to note while interpreting bronchodilator testing are as follows.

1. This test should ideally be performed after withholding respiratory medications based on their duration of action (**Table 1**).

Many protocols are available with differences in bronchodilator used, dose, and mode of delivery without clear evidence supporting one over the other. It will be helpful for clinicians to be familiar with their institutional protocols to accurately interpret and consider modifications if indicated. The various protocols can be found in the 2019 ATS/ERS standard on spirometry.[3]

Box 1
Determination of a bronchodilator response

Bronchodilator response = (post-bronchodilator value (L) – pre-bronchodilator value (L)) × 100 predicted value (L) #
    A change of >10% is considered a significant bronchodilator response.
    #: predicted value should be determined using the appropriate Global Lung Function Initiative (GLI) spirometry equation.
    For example, a 50-year-old man, height 170 cm, has a pre-bronchodilator forced expiratory volume in 1 s (FEV1) of 2.0 L and a post-bronchodilator FEV1 of 2.4 L. The predicted FEV1 is 3.32 L (GLI 2012 "other" equation).

Bronchodilator response = (2.4–2:0) × 100 = 12.1% 3.32
    Therefore, their bronchodilator response is reported as an increase of 12.1% of their predicted FEV1 and classified as a significant response.

Adapted from Stanojevic S, Kaminsky DA, Miller MR, et al. ERS/ATS technical standard on interpretive strategies for routine lung function tests. Eur Respir J 2022; 60: 2101499.

Table 1
Bronchodilator withholding times

Bronchodilator Medication	Withholding Time
SABA (eg, albuterol or salbutamol)	4–6 h
SAMA (eg, ipratropium bromide)	12 h
LABA (eg, formoterol or salmeterol)	24 h
Ultra-LABA (eg, indacaterol, vilanterol, or olodaterol)_	36 h
LAMA (eg, tiotropium, umeclidinium, aclidinium, or glycopyrronium)	36–48 h

Abbreviations: LABA, long acting bronchodilator agent; SABA, short acting bronchodilator agent; SAMA, short acting muscarinic antagonist.
Adapted from Stanojevic S, Kaminsky DA, Miller MR, et al. ERS/ATS technical standard on interpretive strategies for routine lung function tests. Eur Respir J 2022; 60: 2101499.

Sometimes, patients with reversible airway disease may not respond to beta-agonists, so an alternative is inhalation or nebulization of ipratropium bromide aerosol (36 μg), which has a maximal effect at 30 to 45 minutes. In patients who do not respond to standard doses of either drug, a cumulative dose–response protocol can be used, which involves administering aerosol and repeating spirometry at 15-minute intervals until a maximal increase in FEV1 or FVC is attained or limiting symptoms are reached, or a prespecified maximal cumulative dose is reached.

There are a few caveats and key principles to account for in bronchodilatory testing which include.

1. Changes in other indices, such as forced expiratory flow at 25% to 75% of FVC (FEF25%–75%) in response to bronchodilators, are highly variable and should not be used to diagnose asthma.
2. An alternative measure of airflow is measuring parameters such as airway resistance (Raw), airway conductance (Gaw), and specific airway conductance (sGaw). This is measured using body plethysmography, forced oscillometry, and impulse oscillometry but has limited clinical utility. A non-guideline-based cutoff for a significant change in sRaw and sGaw after bronchodilator is 25% to 50% and 40%, respectively, based on pediatric studies.

Finally, it is essential to be aware of the limitations of bronchodilator testing while interpreting this study.

1. First, strict cutoffs for BDR may not account for the variability seen due to age, sex, and baseline lung function. Clinical judgment should be used when you observe a bronchodilator response not meeting American Thoracic Society (ATS) thresholds.
2. Second, a positive BDR is suggestive but not diagnostic of asthma as 35% to 60% of individuals with COPD show a bronchodilator response, more commonly in FVC than FeV1.[2,3]

PEAK FLOW

The peak expiratory flow (PEF or peak flow or peak flow rate) is the maximal rate that a person can exhale during a short maximal expiratory effort after a full inspiration. In patients with asthma, the PEF percent predicted correlates reasonably well with the percent predicted value for the FEV_1 and provides an objective measure of airflow limitation when unavailable spirometry.[4]

PEF measurement using a home peak flow device over a few weeks has been used to objectively demonstrate airflow variability for diagnosing asthma. However, because it relies heavily on patient involvement to perform and document multiple measurements every day, it has a highly variable sensitivity so may not be a reliable or feasible test.[5]

According to the 2023 GINA guidelines, an average daily diurnal variability of greater than 10% by PEF supports a diagnosis of asthma in adults.[1] This requires taking twice a day measurement and is calculated as follows:

Day's highest measurement − day's lowest measurement

mean of day's highest and lowest measurement (averaged over one weak)

ERS 2022 guidelines do not recommend routine peak flow testing to diagnose asthma, reserving it for situations when spirometry and bronchial challenge testing is not possible. PEF may also be helpful for the diagnosis of occupational asthma.[6] The 2007 EPR-3 guidelines concur on using PEF as a monitoring but not a diagnostic tool.[4]

Bronchial Provocation/Challenge Testing

A pathognomic feature of asthma is increased smooth muscle hypertrophy and hyperactivity. Bronchial provocation testing may be indicated to elicit this feature when spirometry fails to demonstrate a variable airflow obstruction in a patient with clinical suspicion of asthma.

This may be important because 25% to 40% of individuals with physician-diagnosed asthma in the community do not have evidence of airway hyperreactivity.[2]

The most used bronchoprovocation test is the methacholine challenge test. Methacholine is a synthetic derivative of the neurotransmitter acetylcholine and directly stimulates muscarinic (M3) receptors on airway smooth muscle when inhaled and causes bronchoconstriction. This test involves exposure to sequential doses (doubling of concentration between doses) of inhaled methacholine (**Fig. 4**).

Inhalation of progressively increasing concentration of methacholine until a positive response is seen or maximum concentration is reached. A positive response is defined as a 20% decrease in FEV1 relative to the value after inhaling a saline control, usually extrapolated between doses if FEV1 falls by more than 20%.

The 2017 ERS standards recommend reporting the minimum dose required inducing a response as the provocative dose (PD20) rather than the concentration (PC20) previously reported. This can be used to grade the degree of bronchial hyper-responsiveness[7] (**Table 2**).

Limitations

1. An abnormal/positive provocation test supports a diagnosis of asthma. Still, it may be seen in other airway diseases such as COPD sarcoidosis, in the setting of allergic rhinitis without lower airway symptoms, or after a recent upper respiratory tract infection or smoking.
2. A normal/negative test provides strong evidence against a diagnosis of asthma but may be falsely negative in exercise-induced asthma, early occupational asthma, or after recent systemic corticosteroid treatment.

In addition to the general contraindications for spirometry and bronchoprovocation testing, relative contraindications specific to methacholine challenge testing include.

1. Pregnancy and nursing mothers
2. Current use of cholinesterase inhibitor medication (eg, for myasthenia gravis).

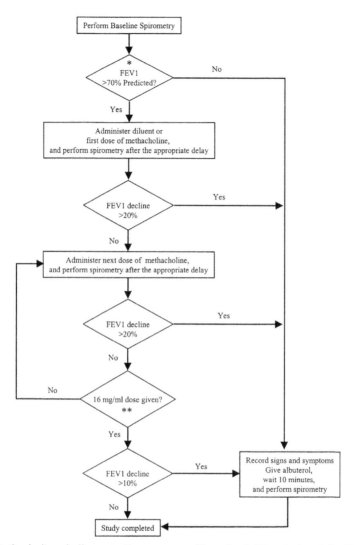

Fig. 4. Methacholine challenge testing sequence (flow chart).*The choice of the FEV1 value considered a contraindication may vary from 60% to 70% of predicted. **The final dose may vary depending on the dosing schedule used. Final doses discussed in this statement are 16, 25, and 32 mg/mL. (*Reprinted with permission* of the American Thoracic Society. Copyright © 2023 American Thoracic Society. All rights reserved. Crapo RO, Casaburi R, Coates AL, et al. Guidelines for methacholine and exercise challenge testing-1999. This official statement of the American Thoracic Society was adopted by the ATS Board of Directors, July 1999. Am J Respir Crit Care Med. 2000;161(1):309-329. The American Journal of Respiratory and Critical Care Medicine is an official journal of the American Thoracic Society.)

Before testing, we typically withhold the medications as shown in **Table 3**.[7]

FRACTIONAL EXHALED NITRIC OXIDE

Nitric oxide can be measured in exhaled breath and correlates with airway inflammation. In individuals with asthma, fractional exhaled nitric oxide (FeNO) may indicate type 2 (T2) bronchial or eosinophilic inflammation in the airway.[8,9]

Table 2
Categorization of airway response to methacholine

PD20 μmol(μg)	PC20 mg.mL-1	Interpretation
>2 (>400)	>16	Normal
0.5–2.0 (100–400)	4–16	Borderline AHR
0.13–0.5 (25–100)	1–4	Mild AHR
0.03–0.13 (6–25)	0.25–1	Moderate AHR
<0.03 (<6)	<0.25	Marked AHR

Abbreviations: AHR, airway hyperresponsiveness; PC20, provocative concentration causing 20% fall in FEV1; PD20, provocative dose causing 20% fall in FEV1.

Per the 2022 guidelines from the National Heart, Lung, and Blood Institute, FeNO can be used when the diagnosis of asthma is uncertain or if spirometry is not feasible but should not be used in isolation. The 2021 ATS guidelines make a conditional recommendation for performing FeNO testing in individuals before starting treatment for asthma in addition to usual care.[4]

It is important to remember that the diagnostic accuracy of the FeNO testing depends on the clinical context, cutoff values used, and multiple other factors, as highlighted in the following (**Table 4**).

1. In corticosteroid-naïve individuals, FeNO less than 20 ppb can rule out asthma (sensitivity of 0.79, specificity of 0.77, and a diagnostic odds ratio of 12.25).
2. Lower FeNO (<25 ppb) is seen in T2 low phenotype asthma, smoking, and corticosteroid use.
3. Higher FeNO levels (>50 ppb) are consistent with elevated T2 inflammation and support a diagnosis of asthma but can also be seen in other conditions with eosinophilic airway inflammation.
4. FeNO levels of 25 to 50 ppb are indeterminate and should be interpreted with caution.

CHALLENGES/PITFALLS OF ASTHMA TESTING

Asthma is a clinical diagnosis without a gold standard diagnostic test. As a result, it is frequently misdiagnosed. The estimates of underdiagnosis of asthma vary widely from as 19% to 73%. For Example, a US study among young adults entering military

Table 3
Medications which may decrease airway hyperresponsiveness and withholding time

Medication	Minimum Time Interval from Last Dose in Hours
Short-acting beta agonists (eg, albuterol)	6
Long-acting beta agonists (eg, salmeterol, formoterol)	36
Ultra-long-acting beta agonist (indacaterol, vilanterol, olodaterol)	48
short acting muscarinic agonists (eg, ipratropium)	12
Long-acting muscarinic agonist (eg, tiotropium, umeclidinium, aclidinium, or glycopyrronium)	>168
Oral theophylline	12–24

Table 4
Interpretations of fractional exhaled nitric oxide test results for asthma diagnosis in nonsmoking individuals not taking corticosteroids

FeNO Level		
<25 ppb (<20 in Children Ages 5–12 y)	25–50 ppb (20–35 in Children Ages 5–12 y)	>50 ppb (>35 in Children Ages 5–12 y)
Recent or current corticosteroid use Alternative diagnoses Phenotype less likely to benefit from ICS Non-eosinophilic asthma COPD Bronchiectasis. CF Vocal cord dysfunction Rhinosinusitis Smoking Obesity	Evaluate in clinical context Consider other diagnoses Consider other factors influencing result Eosinophilic asthma less likely	Eosinophilic airways inflammation likely Phenotype more likely to respond to ICS Allergic asthma Eosinophilic bronchitis

Abbreviation: CF, cystic fibrosis.
Reproduced from Cloutier MM et al 2020 Focused Updates to the Asthma Management Guidelines: A Report from the National Asthma Education and Prevention Program Coordinating Committee Expert Panel Working Group. J Allergy Clin Immunol. 2020 Dec;146(6):1217-1270.

service and undergoing spirometry showed that 30% of participants had a new diagnosis of asthma that had previously been missed.[10,11]

Specific populations are more prone to misdiagnosis. Obese patients are reported to have higher rates of both overdiagnosis and underdiagnosis. Pregnancy excludes patients from bronchoprovocation testing. Elderly patients with multiple comorbidities may also underreport symptoms, and clinicians may attribute them to normal aging, deconditioning, or other comorbidities.

Asthma and COPD are often difficult to distinguish, especially in patients with a smoking history, older patients, or patients with long-standing asthma who have developed persistent, fixed obstruction on spirometry. These two conditions may occur concurrently in asthma–COPD overlap, with worse outcomes than asthma alone. The history, pattern of symptoms, and past spirometry data can help clarify the diagnosis. Diffusing capacity carbon monoxide (DLCO) is often lower in COPD than in asthma.[1]

Owing to its episodic nature, occupational or exercise-induced asthma can also be easily missed as testing may be falsely negative if patient is asymptomatic at the time of testing and had no recent exposure. So, it is essential to have a high index of suspicion and use PEF and bronchoprovocation testing if indicated.

Diagnosis can be challenging in low- and middle-income countries with limited access to lung function testing. The World Health Organization (WHO) recommends evaluating for variable expiratory airflow limitation using PEF instead of relying solely on a syndromic approach.

If treatment with bronchodilator or inhaled corticosteroids is started without confirming a diagnosis this may further confound spirometry, BDR, bronchoprovocation testing, and FeNO. These tests can be falsely negative and incorrectly interpreted to exclude asthma by an inexperienced provider to exclude asthma. If patient's symptoms are well controlled on an inhaled corticosteroids (ICS) medication, reduce their ICS

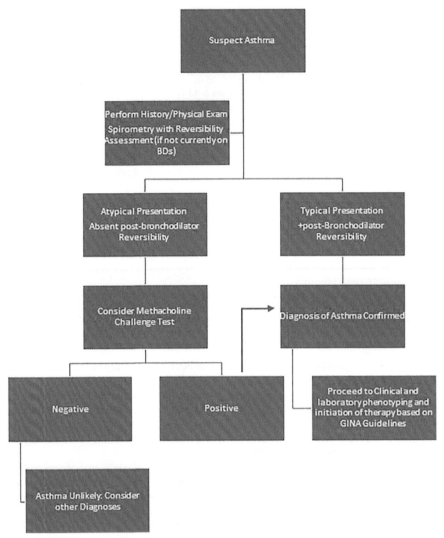

Fig. 5. Suggested algorithm for diagnosing asthma.

dose by 25% to 50%, or stop other maintenance medication, and repeat assessment of symptoms and lung function tests in 2 to 4 weeks. If symptoms increase and variable expiratory airflow obstruction is confirmed, a diagnosis of asthma is confirmed.

However, if symptoms do not worsen and there is still no evidence of variable expiratory airflow limitation, consider ceasing treatment and reassessing in 2 to 3 weeks. Patents may need workup for alternate diagnosis, expert consultation or continued monitoring depending on the response to stop ICS.

If symptoms are poorly controlled or if the patient is at a risk for exacerbation, step down treatment only with expert consultation and close supervision[1]

On the other hand, overdiagnosis is also a pertinent issue in asthma. Studies showed that approximately 30% of patients diagnosed with asthma had no objective evidence to support this diagnosis.[12]

Table 5
Summary of diagnostic testing for asthma

Testing Modality	Interpretation of Positive Finding	Guidelines for Utilization	Notes
Bronchodilator testing	Supports asthma diagnosis in the appropriate clinical context.	Suggest using for initial workup before starting treatment	Reversibility can be seen in other conditions like COPD. Poor sensitivity for asthma (3%–46%), especially in asymptomatic patients. It can be affected by age, sex, and baseline lung function.
FeNO	Suggestive of asthma	It can be used in conjunction with spirometry in the proper clinical context.	Sensitivity and specificity depend on clinical context and cutoff values used. It can be raised in allergic rhinitis, eosinophilic bronchitis, and COPD with eosinophilic phenotype. Low in smokers, non-eosinophilic asthma phenotype, and with corticosteroid use.
Bronchoprovocation testing	Strongly supports asthma diagnosis	Use when clinical suspicion of asthma, but spirometry nondiagnostic	False positives are likely in COPD, cystic fibrosis, sarcoidosis, allergic rhinitis, recent URI, or smoking. False negatives can be seen in exercise-induced asthma, early occupational asthma, or after recent systemic steroid use.
Peak flow	Variability suggestive of asthma	Routine use is not recommended. It can be used to diagnose occupational asthma or when spirometry is unavailable.	Dependent on patient effort, technique, and adherence. Highly variable sensitivity and low accuracy and reliability

SUMMARY

Asthma presents unique challenges to diagnosis due to its episodic nature, wide differential for symptoms, and lack of a standardized approach or gold standard for testing.

Both overdiagnosis and underdiagnosis are associated with inappropriate treatment and potential patient harm. A simplified approach to asthma diagnosis is shown (**Fig. 5**), incorporating the various tests discussed.

There is discordance between the national and international guidelines, but most recommend objective testing with spirometry before treatment, barring clinical urgency (**Table 5**). Bronchial provocation testing should be used where asthma is suspected in which prior investigations have been nondiagnostic. There remains a lack of consensus on the role of FeNO and peak expiratory flow rate (PEFR) testing in diagnosing asthma.

CLINICS CARE POINTS

- Post-bronchodilator spirometry should be considered as a first line test for confirmation of asthma in suspected patients.
- Many patients with suspected asthma may have mimic conditions that should be evaluated when concluding this diagnosis.

DISCLOSURE

This work was supported by NIH (P30027482-14 and 1K08HL1 to GMS).

REFERENCES

1. Venkatesan P. 2023 GINA report for asthma. Lancet Respir Med 2023;11(7):589.
2. Broaddus VC, Ernst JD, King TE, et al. Murray & Nadel's textbook of respiratory medicine. 7th edition. vol 1. New York: Elsevier; 2022.
3. Stanojevic S, Kaminsky DA, Miller MR, et al. ERS/ATS technical standard on interpretive strategies for routine lung function tests. Eur Respir J 2022;60(1):2101499.
4. Cloutier MM, Baptist AP, Baptist AP, et al. 2020 Focused updates to the asthma management guidelines: a report from the national asthma education and prevention program coordinating committee expert panel working group [published correction appears in J Allergy Clin Immunol. 2021 Apr;147(4):1528-1530]. J Allergy Clin Immunol 2020;146(6):1217–70.
5. Goldstein MF, Veza BA, Dunsky EH, et al. Comparisons of peak diurnal expiratory flow variation, postbronchodilator FEV(1) responses, and methacholine inhalation challenges in the evaluation of suspected asthma. Chest 2001;119(4):1001–10.
6. Louis R, Satia I, Ojanguren I, et al. European respiratory society guidelines for the diagnosis of asthma in adults [published online ahead of print, 2022 Feb 15]. Eur Respir J 2022;2101585. https://doi.org/10.1183/13993003.01585-2021.
7. Coates AL, Wanger J, Cockcroft DW, et al. ERS technical standard on bronchial challenge testing: general considerations and performance of methacholine challenge tests. Eur Respir J 2017;49(5):1601526.
8. Dweik RA, Boggs PB, Erzurum SC, et al. An official ATS clinical practice guideline: interpretation of exhaled nitric oxide levels (FENO) for clinical applications. Am J Respir Crit Care Med 2011;184(5):602–15.

9. Khatri SB, Iaccarino JM, Barochia A, et al. Use of fractional exhaled nitric oxide to guide the treatment of asthma: an official American thoracic society clinical practice guideline. Am J Respir Crit Care Med 2021;204(10):e97–109.

10. Nolte H, Nepper-Christensen S, Backer V. Unawareness and undertreatment of asthma and allergic rhinitis in a general population. Respir Med 2006;100(2): 354–62.

11. De Marco R, Cerveri I, Bugiani M, et al. An undetected burden of asthma in Italy: the relationship between clinical and epidemiological diagnosis of asthma. Eur Respir J 1998;11(3):599–605.

12. Kavanagh J, Jackson DJ, Kent BD. Over- and under-diagnosis in asthma. Breathe 2019;15(1):e20–7.

Asthma Management Considerations for the Otolaryngologist: Current Therapies

Dhanya Asokumar, BS, Amarbir S. Gill, MD*

KEYWORDS

• Asthma • Chronic rhinosinusitis • Treatment • Management • Multidisciplinary

KEY POINTS

- Asthma is frequently comorbid with chronic rhinosinusitis (CRS) and should be evaluated for in the presence of CRS. Management of comorbid respiratory causes such as CRS usually leads to improved asthma outcomes.
- The preferred stepwise approach to pharmacologic intervention for asthma includes the following: inhaled corticosteroid (ICS)-formoterol as needed → low-dose ICS-formoterol maintenance → medium-dose ICS-formoterol → consider adding long-acting muscarinic antagonist, biologic, or replacing with high-dose formoterol.
- Given the significant adverse effects of oral corticosteroids, they should be used judiciously, with the number of courses prescribed monitored closely, and patients should be counseled on the side effect profile.

INTRODUCTION

Asthma is a disease characterized by underlying airway inflammation, bronchial hyperresponsiveness, and reversible airflow obstruction.[1,2] Globally, asthma is the 28th leading cause of burden of disease, afflicting more than 26 million Americans,[3] and resulting in an annual economic burden of US$80 billion.[4]

As specialists in the upper airways, otolaryngology providers are in a unique position to manage certain comorbid conditions that frequently occur alongside asthma, such as chronic rhinosinusitis (CRS). CRS can increase the risk of asthma-related exacerbations and emergency department visits, contribute to worse disease-specific quality of life (QOL), and increase asthma-related medication usage.[5,6] Greater than two-thirds of people with asthma have symptoms of rhinosinusitis and up to 45% of

Department of Otolaryngology – Head and Neck Surgery, University of Michigan, Ann Arbor, MI, USA
* Corresponding author. 1500 East Medical Center Dr. 1904 TC, SPC 5312, Ann Arbor, MI 48109.
E-mail address: asingill@med.umich.edu

Otolaryngol Clin N Am 57 (2024) 215–224
https://doi.org/10.1016/j.otc.2023.10.001
0030-6665/24/© 2023 Elsevier Inc. All rights reserved.

individuals with asthma have comorbid CRS (chronic rhinosinusitis with asthma [CRSwA]; **Fig. 1**).[7]

EPIDEMIOLOGY
Disease Risk Factors

According to the Global Strategy for Asthma Management and Prevention (GINA) guidelines, acute asthma exacerbations are defined as "episodes of progressive increase in shortness of breath, cough, wheezing, or chest tightness, or some combination of these symptoms, accompanied by decreases in expiratory airflow that can be quantified by measurement of lung function."[8,9] There are several factors associated with an increased risk of acute exacerbations and poor asthma outcomes; they can be categorized as modifiable or nonmodifiable (**Table 1**).[8] Even if individuals exhibit few asthma symptoms, these risk factors increase the risk of exacerbations.[8] The literature has shown that CRS is an independent risk factor for asthma exacerbations and more difficult-to-control asthma.[10] Patients with CRS are also at an increased risk for developing comorbid asthma.[11] Moreover, data demonstrate that endoscopic sinus surgery (ESS) for the management of CRS can lead to improved asthma control, less asthma-related health-care utilization, and a reduction in asthma-specific medication usage in the immediate postoperative period.[5] Similarly, ESS can improve both sinonasal-specific and asthma-specific QOL outcomes during this timeframe.[5]

Prevention

As a heterogenous and complex disease, asthma is influenced by a multitude of factors, including genetic and environmental features. Primary prevention refers to interventions that are implemented before the development of disease; in the case of asthma, primary prevention targets children and involves counseling on the avoidance of tobacco smoke exposure and encouraging vaginal births.[8] There is no strong

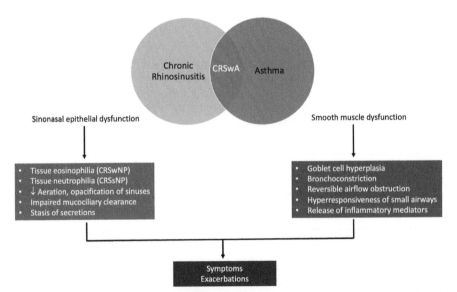

Fig. 1. Asthma and chronic rhinosinusitis unified airway pathophysiology. CRSsNP, chronic rhinosinusitis without nasal polyps; CRSwA, chronic rhinosinusitis with asthma; CRSwNP, chronic rhinosinusitis with nasal polyps.

Table 1			
Risk factors for exacerbations and poor asthma outcomes independent of medication adherence			
Modifiable Risk Factors	**Nonmodifiable Risk Factors**	**Otolaryngologic Comorbidities**	**Other Comorbidities**
Smoking	$\geq$1 exacerbation in last 12 mos	Chronic rhinosinusitis	Obesity
Environmental exposures	Low FEV_1	Allergic rhinitis	COPD
Allergen exposures	Blood eosinophilia	AERD	Depression
Medications (β-blockers, NSAIDs, high SABA usage related side-effects)	Family history	Nasal polyposis	Anxiety
	Genetics		Atopic dermatitis
Anxiety or psychological difficulties			GERD
Socioeconomic status			Obstructive sleep apnea
			Pregnancy

Abbreviations: AERD, aspirin exacerbated respiratory disease; COPD, chronic obstructive pulmonary disease; FEV_1, forced expiratory volume; GERD, gastroesophageal reflux disease; LAMA, long-acting muscarinic antagonist; NSAIDS, nonsteroidal anti-inflammatory drugs; OCS, oral corticosteroids; SABA, short-acting-β-agonist; β-blockers, Beta-blockers.
Adapted from Global Initiative for Asthma. Global Strategy for Asthma Management and Prevention, 2023 (GINA, 2023).

evidence to support that dietary changes, weight loss, or early-life exposure to allergens are effective in primary prevention.[8] Especially in the context of multiple risk factors, triggers are important to identify on an individual level to achieve prevention and intervention at the early stages.

Triggers for asthma include the following:[7]

- Allergens
- Irritants
- History of aspirin sensitivity or other cyclooxygenase 1-inhibiting nonsteroidal anti-inflammatory drug sensitivity
- Bacterial or viral infections

Chronic Rhinosinusitis Management

Similarly, prevention and early treatment of comorbid upper airway disease is important to manage disease severity, QOL, and mortality. Primary prevention of CRS has focused on eliminating risk factors for the disease, including avoiding environmental factors such as tobacco and occupational toxins.[12] Secondary and tertiary prevention focus on early detection and treatment, and minimization of further progression of disease, respectively. Patient counseling is essential for secondary and tertiary prevention and targets early detection, early pharmacologic/surgical intervention, and maximization of QOL.[9]

PHARMACOLOGIC THERAPEUTICS

As outlined by the GINA 2023 guidelines, asthma management should include symptom control, minimizing risk of exacerbations and mortality, addressing comorbidities, and managing patient priorities and goals.[8] Managing comorbidities of asthma is important to improve factors such as QOL and symptomatic exacerbations. Specific to CRS, individuals with asthma and comorbid respiratory disease have demonstrated improvements in lower airway symptoms when sinonasal symptoms are well managed.[8] The following sections focus on conventional (nonbiologic) therapies for the management of asthma (**Fig. 2**).

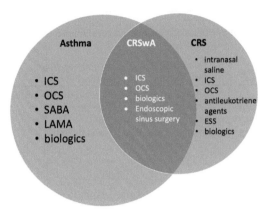

Fig. 2. Pharmacologic therapeutic considerations for patients with asthma, CRS, and CRSwA. CRS, chronic rhinosinusitis; CRSwA, chronic rhinosinusitis with asthma; ESS, endoscopic sinus surgery; ICS, inhaled corticosteroids; LAMA, long-acting muscarinic antagonist; OCS, oral corticosteroids; SABA, short-acting-beta-agonist.

Asthma treatment should be managed using a stepwise approach that is initiated as soon as the asthma diagnosis is made (**Fig. 3**). If a patient demonstrates exacerbations/symptoms despite controller treatment, the provider should assess factors that can lead to suboptimal outcomes before escalating treatment. These factors include incorrect inhaler techniques, nonadherence to medication, exposure to irritants (eg, pollutants, allergens, and tobacco smoke), incorrect diagnosis, and comorbidities contributing to respiratory symptoms.[8] Patients who have maintained

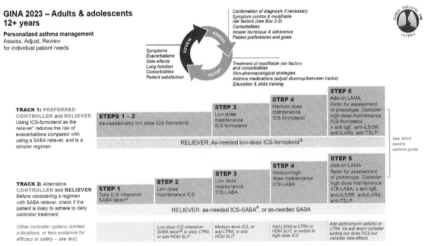

Fig. 3. Summary of initial pharmacologic treatment recommendations based on GINA recommendations for asthma patients. Interventions following first-line therapeutics are used if condition is medically recalcitrant. AIR, anti-inflammatory reliever; ICS, inhaled corticosteroids; LABA, long-acting-β-agonist; LAMA, long-acting muscarinic antagonist; OCS, oral corticosteroids; SABA, short-acting-β-agonist. [a]Anti-inflammatory reliever (AIR) (*Reproduced with written permission from* © 2023, Global Initiative for Asthma, available from ginasthma.org, published in Fontana, WI, USA)

adequate symptom control using the proposed stepwise approach for 2 to 3 months may adjust treatment in a step-down method to find the minimum necessary treatment to achieve good symptom control.[8]

Inhaled Corticosteroids

The mainstay of treatment of individuals with asthma is inhaled corticosteroid (ICS) medication to control symptoms and reduce symptom exacerbations.[8] Data demonstrate that ICS therapy started soon after the development of symptoms leads to better outcomes than if ICS therapy is initiated when symptoms have been present for more than 2 years.[13] In patients with minimal symptoms (<4 d/wk with no exacerbations in last 12 months) and no risk factors for exacerbations, the recommendation is to use a low-dose ICS-formoterol and a long-acting-β-agonist (LABA), as needed for symptom control (see **Fig. 3**).[8] Budesonide or beclomethasone are effective low-dose ICSs used in combination with formoterol for this purpose.[8,14] In the case of persistent symptoms, including symptoms leading to awakenings at night and continued evidence of poor pulmonary function, treatment should be escalated to low-dose maintenance daily ICS-formoterol and then to medium-dose daily ICS-formoterol, if needed. If acute exacerbations or severe, uncontrolled symptoms were present initially, medium-dose ICS-formoterol maintenance could be initiated from the start, without a trial of low-dose ICS-formoterol.[8] Judicious, infrequent, and short courses of oral corticosteroids (OCSs) may be considered for severe, uncontrolled exacerbations. Continued poor control should trigger consideration of an add-on long-acting muscarinic antagonist (LAMA), as well as further escalation to high-dose ICS-formoterol ± biologic medication.[8]

Although short-acting-β-agonists (SABAs), such as albuterol, have been historically used as the sole rescue option for individuals with asthma, it has been demonstrated that ICS-formoterol reduces exacerbations more than SABA relievers and is the preferred pathway. Moreover, studies have shown that SABA-alone treatment increases the risk for asthma-related exacerbations and mortality.[8] Despite quick symptom control, patients with SABA-only treatment have decreased lung function, poorer outcomes, and more asthma-related emergencies compared with patients with ICS treatment.[8] Nevertheless, according to the GINA guidelines, an alternative treatment pathway using SABA or ICS-SABA as a reliever medication is an option for individuals with stable disease who demonstrate good adherence to their current regimen and have not had any recent exacerbations (see **Fig. 3**).[15] On this pathway, it is recommended that ICS be taken anytime SABA is used. Treatment on this pathway up can be escalated to low-dose maintenance ICS if symptoms persist for more than 2 times per month.[8] Escalation to a low-dose dual ICS-LABA therapy (eg, budesonide, ciclesonide, and mometasone) is recommended if the individual has symptoms on most days or waking due to asthma symptoms.[8] If symptoms continue to interfere with QOL, or there is evidence of continued poor pulmonary function, treatment should be escalated to medium-dose or high-dose maintenance ICS-LABA treatment, and judicious use of OCS as needed for exacerbations.[8] Patients with severe asthma recalcitrant to the aforementioned regimens may need an add-on LAMA, high-dose maintenance of ICS-LABA and/or biologic medication.[8]

β-Agonists

LABAs decrease acetylcholine release and stimulate smooth muscle relaxation and bronchodilation. Their efficacy is improved when used in combination with ICS, which suppresses proinflammatory transcription factors.[16] Examples of approved ICS-LABA combinations include fluticasone furoate-vilanterol, fluticasone propionate-salmeterol, mometasone-formoterol, and budesonide-formoterol.[8,17] ICS-formoterol (budesonide/beclomethasone-formoterol) is a rapid onset LABA and the preferred first-line treatment of people with asthma. This combination has reduced severe exacerbations by up to 64% compared with SABA when used as needed.[8] ICS-LABA treatment can also improve symptom control in other respiratory diseases, such as asthma chronic obstructive pulmonary disease (COPD) overlap syndrome (ACOS), and is the preferred therapeutic option for this disease.[18]

Muscarinic Antagonists

LAMAs, such as tiotropium, can be used as an additional inhaler for uncontrolled asthma. It should be considered after escalating treatment to medium-dose/high-dose ICS-LABA treatment. Tiotropium can improve lung function and decrease the risk of severe exacerbations[8]; however, asthma-specific symptoms do not seem to improve significantly. LAMAs should not be added-on before medium-dose ICS-LABAs have been tried because there is no evidence to support ICS-LAMA usage over ICS-LABAs as monotherapy.[8] Although LAMAs reduce asthma-related exacerbations and mortality, they should not be used without ICS therapy because this can increase the risk of severe exacerbations. A single clinical trial suggested that asthma-related hospitalizations were greater in patients on ICS-tiotropium compared with the ICS-LABA group.[19] ICS-LABA-LAMA triple therapy has also been shown to improve lung function in other lower airway diseases, such as ACOS and COPD, although more studies are needed to investigate whether this also translates into improved symptom control.[20,21] The available triple-therapy combinations include beclomethasone-formoterol-glycopyrronium, fluticasone furoate-vilanterol-umeclindium, and mometasone-indacaterol-glycopyrronium.[8]

Oral Corticosteroids

OCSs, such as prednisone or prednisolone, are highly effective at managing asthma exacerbations; however, they should be used sparingly because of a significant side effect profile. OCS should only be used in individuals with poor symptom control and frequent exacerbations as a last resort.[8] The possibility of a severe exacerbation is considered when an individual is not responding to therapeutics for 2 days, or the forced expiratory volume (FEV_1) is less than 60% predicted. Long-term OCS usage can lead to osteoporosis, cataracts, depression, anxiety, adrenal suppression, ischemic heart disease, and hypertension.[22,23] Specifically, patients using more than 4 OCS courses have a significantly higher risk of developing these adverse side effects within the first year of treatment.[24] Furthermore, continued use during multiple years has proven to be additive.[24]

Alarmingly, one study found that 21% of patients with asthma with regular OCS usage died compared with 5.5% and 4.5% of periodic and non-OCS users, respectively.[23] Despite the evident OCS-related mortality and risks, 40% to 60% of people with severe asthma use long-term OCS.[25] Studies have shown that the toxic threshold dose is 1000 mg prednisolone during a lifetime (eg, 5 OCS courses of 40 mg/5 d).[24] Patients with high OCS exposure above this are at a higher risk of developing osteoporosis, adrenal insufficiency, renal impairments, cerebrovascular disease, and infections. Furthermore, the health-care costs of people with severe asthma using OCS are 40% higher than those not using OCS.[24]

A study assessing perspectives of patients with severe asthma on their therapeutic management concluded that patients are concerned and want more information on OCS side effects than what is given to them from their providers, highlighting the importance of physician counseling for patients considering OCS therapeutics.[26]

Montelukast

If a low-dose ICS is not available for step 2 or 3 escalations (see **Fig. 3**), leukotriene receptor antagonists may be used; however, they are less effective than ICS or LABAs in preventing exacerbation and have a boxed Food and Drug Administration warning for the associated neuropsychiatric side effects.[8] Nevertheless, LRTAs are still recommended as add-on treatments, especially if biologic agents are not available for difficult-to-treat and severe asthma (ie, uncontrolled disease despite high ICS-LABA).[8] Montelukast has been shown to intermittently benefit patients with asthma patients with nasal polyposis; however, it has not been shown to improve their lung function.[27,28]

Immunotherapy

When allergies contribute significantly to asthma exacerbations, or when a comorbidity such as allergic rhinoconjunctivitis is present, allergen-specific immunotherapy may be considered. Sublingual allergen immunotherapy (SLIT) is recommended for individuals with allergic rhinitis, dust sensitization, or poor asthma control despite ICS usage.[8] Subcutaneous immunotherapy (SCIT) is associated with improvement in symptoms, airway hyperresponsiveness, and less medication requirements, whereas SLIT shows increased periods between exacerbations during ICS therapy reduction. Because of the demanding requirements of completing SCIT and SLIT therapy (cost, time, and adverse effects), these immunotherapies are highly dependent on individual priorities and capacity for benefits.[8]

Intranasal Corticosteroids

Strong research evidence shows that topical intranasal corticosteroids (INCSs) and nasal saline irrigations are an effective first-line treatment for the management of sinonasal symptoms in CRS and chronic rhinosinusitis with asthma (CRSwA). INCS reduces inflammation and improves nasal symptoms, such as anosmia and nasal blockage, and has a limited side effect profile.[29] Although INCSs have been shown to improve sinonasal outcomes in patients with CRS, there are no studies that have investigated the effect on lung function or asthma control.[9]

NONPHARMACOLOGICAL THERAPEUTICS
Avoidance and Modifiable Risk Factors

Although pharmacologic treatments have been found to be effective for asthma, other interventions may assist in improving symptom control and exacerbations. It is recommended that physicians counsel patients to stop smoking and minimize environmental tobacco exposure (ETS), engage in physical activity, avoid occupational exposures, and consume healthy diets.[8] The former can prevent bronchoconstriction, whereas eliminating occupational sensitizers (eg, industrial settings and latex gloves), consuming fruit and vegetables, and engaging in breathing exercise have been shown to improve QOL and reduce stress.[8]

There is weak evidence to support prescribing β-blockers only with close supervision and/or avoiding their prescription in individuals with asthma. There is strong evidence to support the avoidance of aspirin and nonsteroidal anti-inflammatory drugs (NSAIDs) if there is a history of adverse reactions to them.[8]

It is currently not recommended that individuals with asthma engage in avoidance of indoor allergens (eg, dust mites, pest rodents, and furry pets) because it has not been shown to improve outcomes.[8] A weak evidence shows that avoidance of outdoor allergens improves clinical outcomes of patients with asthma.[8]

DISCUSSION

Although there are stepwise interventions based on daily symptoms and exacerbations, further studies are needed to clearly define mild asthma and to assess the meaning of "symptom control" achieved from treatments.[8] To this end, the term "mild asthma" should be avoided in clinical settings because of the heterogeneity in definitions, whereas severe asthma and difficult-to-treat asthma definitions are well supported. The mainstay of treatment of individuals with asthma is ICS medication with a shift to ICS-formoterol over SABA when considering a reliever among individuals with asthma. From here, the GINA guidelines outline a stepwise escalation of treatment with limited and judicious use of OCS for severe, uncontrolled exacerbations. Evidence does not support allergen avoidance indoors for improvement of asthma symptoms, and further studies are needed to clarify the utility of SLIT and SCIT allergen immunotherapy in this cohort of individuals.

SUMMARY

Management of patients with unified airway disease should incorporate a multidisciplinary approach utilizing both otolaryngologists and asthma specialists. Given the serious side effects and long-term sequalae, OCS should be used sparingly and patients should be counseled on the side effects of OCS usage, with the number of courses prescribed monitored closely.

CLINICS CARE POINTS

- Given their highly comorbid nature, patients with CRS should be evaluated for the presence of asthma.
- The following is the preferred stepwise pharmacologic intervention for individuals with asthma: ICS-formoterol as needed → low-dose ICS-formoterol maintenance → medium-dose ICS-formoterol → add LAMA, and/or replacing with high-dose formoterol, consider adding biologic.
- Nonpharmacologic interventions for asthma:
  ○ Counsel patients on smoking cessation, minimize ETS exposure, engage in physical activity, avoid occupational exposures, and consume healthy diets.
  ○ Identify and eliminate occupational sensitizers.

DISCLOSURE

The authors have nothing to disclose.

REFERENCES

1. Brutsche MH, Downs SH, Schindler C, et al. Bronchial hyperresponsiveness and the development of asthma and COPD in asymptomatic individuals: SAPALDIA cohort study. Thorax 2006;61(8):671–7.
2. Bakakos A, Vogli S, Dimakou K, et al. Asthma with Fixed Airflow Obstruction: From Fixed to Personalized Approach. J Pers Med 2022;12(3):333. Published 2022 Feb 23.
3. Dharmage SC, Perret JL, Custovic A. Epidemiology of Asthma in Children and Adults. Front Pediatr 2019;7:246.
4. Centers for Disease Control and Prevention. National Vital. Statistics Reports 2013;61(4).

5. Tiotiu A, Plavec D, Novakova S, et al. Current opinions for the management of asthma associated with ear, nose and throat comorbidities. Eur Respir Rev 2018;27(150):180056. Published 2018 Nov 21.
6. Gleadhill C, Speth MM, Gengler I, et al. Chronic rhinosinusitis disease burden is associated with asthma-related emergency department usage. Eur Arch Oto-Rhino-Laryngol 2020;278(1):93–9.
7. Massoth L, Anderson C, McKinney KA. Asthma and Chronic Rhinosinusitis: Diagnosis and Medical Management. Medical Sciences 2019;7(4):53.
8. Global Initiative for Ashtma, Global Strategy for asthma management and prevention 2023, GINA; Fontana, WI, Available at: ginasthma.org. 2023.
9. Fuhlbrigge A, Peden D, Apter AJ, et al. Asthma outcomes: exacerbations. J Allergy Clin Immunol 2012;129(3 Suppl):S34–48.
10. Gill AS, Alt JA, Detwiller KY, et al. Management paradigms for chronic rhinosinusitis in individuals with asthma: An evidence-based review with recommendations. Int Forum Allergy Rhinol 2022. https://doi.org/10.1002/alr.23130.
11. Hirsch AG, Yan XS, Sundaresan AS, et al. Five-year risk of incident disease following a diagnosis of chronic rhinosinusitis. Allergy 2015;70(12):1613–21.
12. Reh DD, Higgins TS, Smith TL. Impact of tobacco smoke on chronic rhinosinusitis: a review of the literature. Int Forum Allergy Rhinol 2012;2(5):362–9.
13. Selroos O, Pietinalho A, Löfroos AB, et al. Effect of early vs late intervention with inhaled corticosteroids in asthma. Chest 1995;108(5):1228–34.
14. Papi A, Paggiaro PL, Nicolini G, et al, Inhaled Combination Asthma Treatment versus SYmbicort ICAT SY Study Group. Inhaled Combination Asthma Treatment versus Symbicort (ICAT SY) Study Group. Beclomethasone/formoterol versus budesonide/formoterol combination therapy in asthma. Eur Respir J 2007;29(4):682–9.
15. Beasley R, Bruce P, Houghton C, et al. The ICS/Formoterol Reliever Therapy Regimen in Asthma: A Review. J Allergy Clin Immunol Pract 2023;11(3):762–72.e1.
16. Newton R, Giembycz MA. Understanding how long-acting β2 -adrenoceptor agonists enhance the clinical efficacy of inhaled corticosteroids in asthma - an update. Br J Pharmacol 2016;173(24):3405–30.
17. Dave Hoang. Laba-ICS combination. Minnesota Department of Human Services; 2018. Available at: https://mn.gov/dhs/partners-and-providers/policies-procedures/minnesota-health-care-programs/provider/types/rx/pa-criteria/laba-ics-combination.jsp. Accessed July 13, 2023.
18. Oh YM. Is the Combination of ICS and LABA, a Therapeutic Option for COPD, Fading Away? Tuberc Respir Dis 2017;80(1):93–4. https://doi.org/10.4046/trd.2017.80.1.93.
19. Wechsler ME, Yawn BP, Fuhlbrigge AL, et al. Anticholinergic vs Long-Acting β-Agonist in Combination With Inhaled Corticosteroids in Black Adults With Asthma: The BELT Randomized Clinical Trial. JAMA 2015;314(16):1720–30.
20. Ishiura Y, Fujimura M, Ohkura N, et al. Effect of triple therapy in patients with asthma-COPD overlap. Int J Clin Pharmacol Ther 2019;57(8):384–92.
21. Qin J, Wang G, Han D. Benefits of LAMA in patients with asthma-COPD overlap: A systematic review and meta-analysis. Clin Immunol 2022;237:108986.
22. Foster JM, McDonald VM, Guo M, et al. "I have lost in every facet of my life": the hidden burden of severe asthma. Eur Respir J 2017;50(3):1700765.
23. Ekström M, Nwaru BI, Hasvold P, et al. Oral corticosteroid use, morbidity and mortality in asthma: A nationwide prospective cohort study in Sweden. Allergy

2019;74(11):2181–90 [published correction appears in Allergy. 2020;75(8): 2148-2148].

24. Blakey J, Chung LP, McDonald VM, et al. Oral corticosteroids stewardship for asthma in adults and adolescents: A position paper from the Thoracic Society of Australia and New Zealand. Respirology 2021;26(12):1112–30.

25. Haughney J, Winders T, Holmes S, et al. A Charter to Fundamentally Change the Role of Oral Corticosteroids in the Management of Asthma. Adv Ther 2023;40(6): 2577–94.

26. Cooper V, Metcalf L, Versnel J, et al. Patient-reported side effects, concerns and adherence to corticosteroid treatment for asthma, and comparison with physician estimates of side-effect prevalence: a UK-wide, cross-sectional study. NPJ Prim Care Respir Med 2015;25:15026.

27. Kieff DA, Busaba NY. Efficacy of montelukast in the treatment of nasal polyposis. Ann Otol Rhinol Laryngol 2005;114(12):941–5.

28. Schäper C, Noga O, Koch B, et al. Anti-inflammatory properties of montelukast, a leukotriene receptor antagonist in patients with asthma and nasal polyposis. J Investig Allergol Clin Immunol 2011;21(1):51–8.

29. Chong LY, Head K, Hopkins C, et al. Different types of intranasal steroids for chronic rhinosinusitis. Cochrane Database Syst Rev 2016;4(4):CD011993.

Current and Novel Biologic Therapies for Patients with Asthma and Nasal Polyps

Hanna K. Mandl, BS[a], Jessa E. Miller, MD[b],
Daniel M. Beswick, MD[b],*

KEYWORDS

- Biologics • Asthma • Nasal polyps • Chronic rhinosinusitis
- Th2-mediated inflammation • Endotypes • Phenotypes

KEY POINTS

- Biologic agents are an expanding therapeutic option for the management of refractory asthma and nasal polyps.
- The currently Food and Drug Administration (FDA)-approved biologic agents are monoclonal antibodies, which target Th2-mediated inflammation.
- Categorizing asthma and nasal polyps into specific endotypes and phenotypes permits individualized, targeted treatment with biologic agents.
- There are currently six FDA-approved biologics to treat asthma, three of which are also approved for nasal polyps.

INTRODUCTION

Asthma and nasal polyps (NPs) are common diseases that often coexist and share overlapping pathogenesis. Asthma affects nearly 300 million individuals worldwide and consists of chronic airway inflammation, bronchial hyperresponsiveness, mucus production, and airflow obstruction.[1–3]

Chronic rhinosinusitis (CRS) is prevalent and occurs in approximately 2% to 27% of the general population.[4–10] CRS is a heterogeneous process that consists of various phenotypes and endotypes.[11] The two primary phenotypes include CRS with NPs (CRSwNP) and CRS without NPs.[11] NPs are benign inflammatory growths from the sinonasal mucosa and are estimated to occur in approximately 2% to 4% of the general population.[10,12–15] Numerous conditions can be associated with CRSwNP,

[a] University of California, Los Angeles, David Geffen School of Medicine, Los Angeles, CA, USA;
[b] Department of Otolaryngology–Head and Neck Surgery, University of California, Los Angeles, Los Angeles, CA, USA
* Corresponding author. Department of Head and Neck Surgery, University of California, Los Angeles, 10833 Le Conte Avenue, CHS 62-235, Los Angeles, CA 90095-1624.
E-mail address: dbeswick@mednet.ucla.edu

Otolaryngol Clin N Am 57 (2024) 225–242
https://doi.org/10.1016/j.otc.2023.08.006
0030-6665/24/© 2023 Elsevier Inc. All rights reserved.

including allergic fungal sinusitis, aspirin-exacerbated respiratory disease, cystic fibrosis, eosinophilic granulomatosis with polyangiitis, and central compartment atopic disease, among others.

In contrast to phenotypes, which refer to observable clinical traits, endotypes describe a subtype of disease that is defined by a specific molecular mechanism or treatment response.[11,16] The asthma endotypes include Th2-high (eosinophilic) and Th2-low (non-eosinophilic) processes.[2,17] Th2 inflammation plays a significant role in asthma and is mediated by cytokines such as interleukin (IL)-4, IL-5, and IL-13.[17,18] Elevated levels of fractional exhaled nitric oxide (FE_{NO}), immunoglobulin (Ig) E, and other biomarkers may be observed and contribute to mucus secretion, bronchial hyperresponsiveness, airway remodeling, and other features of asthma.[17,19]

Sinonasal endotypes refer to distinct immunologic pathways that are associated with CRS and are determined by biomarkers and gene expression.[10,20] Recent research efforts have focused on defining CRS endotypes based on nasal mucus and tissue biomarkers.[10,11,21–24] Although research on the optimal biomarkers for endotyping is ongoing, current research suggests that Th1, Th2, and Th17 markers play an important role in the pathophysiology of CRS. CRSwNP is typically considered a type 2 eosinophilic inflammatory response in North American and European populations.[20,25]

The unified airway theory refers to the fact that the upper and lower airways are connected anatomically and physiologically.[26–29] Pathologies affecting the upper and lower airways often share a similar immunologic response; specifically, type 2 immune reactions. Because of the unified airway theory, there has been a recent shift in treatment paradigms for individuals with diseases of the upper and lower airways, such as CRSwNP and asthma, respectively. With the development of biologic medications, it is now possible to treat individuals with comorbid asthma and CRSwNP with a single systemic therapy.

Owing to the increased understanding of the complex mechanisms underlying asthma and CRSwNP, targeted monoclonal antibodies (mAb) have been developed.[30] This review aims to discuss the Food and Drug Administration (FDA)-approved biologic agents for the treatment of asthma and CRSwNP and to highlight the current challenges and future directions for these biologic medications.

DISCUSSION
Biological Management of Asthma

Biologic agents serve as an adjunctive treatment in asthma and primarily target type 2 inflammation.[3] Here, the authors discuss the mechanism, indications, clinical trials, administration, side effects, treatment response, and guidelines for use of these biologic agents in the treatment of asthma (**Table 1**).

Immunoglobulin E

IgE has a known role in allergies and is the hallmark of type 1 hypersensitivity reactions.[31] IgE and mast cells are concentrated in mucosal tissues and are activated on exposure to an allergen.[31,32] In sensitized individuals, an immediate allergic hypersensitivity response occurs, which is mediated by a complex formation between IgE and its high-affinity receptors on mast cells.[32] This results in mast cell degranulation, release of cytokines and chemokines, and recruitment of pro-inflammatory cells.[31,32] IgE-sensitized antigen-presenting cells are also activated to induce additional IgE production by B cells.[32] These processes increase activation and production of IgE, contributing to overt symptoms in allergic asthma and CRSwNP.[31,32]

Table 1
Summary of biologic medications approved for asthma and chronic rhinosinusitis with nasal polyposis

Biologic Agent	Target	Approved for	Approval Date	Dose	Route of Admin.	Eligibility Criteria	Side Effects
Omalizumab	IgE	Moderate to severe persistent asthma; CRSwNPs; CSU[43]	Asthma: 2003[3,34] CRSwNP: 2020[82]	Asthma: 75–375 mg every 2–4 wk[32] CRSwNP: 75–600 mg every 2–4 wk[82]	SC[33]	Asthma: Positive skin testing result to aeroallergen; poorly controlled symptoms with ICS[32] CRSwNP: Inadequate response to INCS[83]	Rash, diarrhea, nausea, vomiting, epistaxis, menorrhagia, hematoma, injection-site reactions, fatigue, paresthesia, anaphylaxis[33,36,113–116]
Mepolizumab	IL-5	Severe eosinophilic asthma; CRSwNPs; eosinophilic granulomatosis with polyangiitis (Churg–Strauss syndrome); hypereosinophilic syndrome (HES)[38,41,42]	Asthma: 2015[36,42] CRSwNP: 2021[81]	Asthma: 100 mg dose every 4 wk, for min 4 mo of treatment for adults[36,42] CRSwNP: 100 mg every 4 wk[117]	SC[36,42]	Asthma: ≥2 asthma exacerbations in the past year or long-term oral corticosteroid use; blood eosinophils >150 cells/µL within 6 wk of initial dosing or ≥ 300 cells/µL within 12 mo of initial dosing[36,42] CRSwNP: Inadequate response to INCS[84]	Injection-site reactions, headache[36,42,50]
Reslizumab	IL-5	Severe eosinophilic asthma[38,49]	Asthma: 2016[36,43]	Asthma: 3 mg/kg every 4 wk[36,43]	IV, given over 20–50 min[36,43]	Asthma: One asthma exacerbation in the prior year and an eosinophil count ≥ 400 cells/µL[36,42,49]	Headache, nasopharyngitis, infusion-site reactions, hypersensitivity reactions, fatigue, pharyngolaryngeal pain, anaphylaxis[36]

(continued on next page)

Table 1
(continued)

Biologic Agent	Target	Approved for	Approval Date	Dose	Route of Admin.	Eligibility Criteria	Side Effects
Benralizumab	IL-5	Severe eosinophilic asthma[36,42]	Asthma: 2017[38,100]	Asthma: 30 mg every 4 wk for the first 3 doses; 30 mg every 8 wk thereafter[36]	SC[36]	Asthma: Eosinophil count $\geq$ 300 cells/μL[36,42]	Nasopharyngitis, worsening asthma[36,100]
Dupilumab	IL-3, IL-14	Moderate to severe eosinophilic asthma or OCS-dependent asthma; CRSwNPs; AD; EoE; PN[19,42]	Asthma: 2018[18] CRSwNP: 2017[85]	Asthma: Once every 2 wk or once every 4 wk, depending on age; for adults, 400 mg or 600 mg loading dose, with 200 mg or 300 mg maintenance doses thereafter; higher doses for OCS-dependent asthma[65] CRSwNP: 300 mg every other week[118]	SC[65]	Asthma: Patients 6 y or older with moderate to severe eosinophilic asthma or OCS-dependent asthma[18,65] CRSwNP: Inadequately controlled CRSwNP[86]	Injection-site reactions, nasopharyngitis, bronchitis, sinusitis, nausea, headache, eosinophilia[18,19]
Tezepelumab	TSLP	Severe uncontrolled asthma[68]	Asthma: 2021[68]	Asthma: 210 mg once every 4 wk[68]	SC[68]	Asthma: Patients with uncontrolled asthma despite treatment with both high-dose ICS and an additional maintenance medication[68]	Headache, elevated creatine phosphokinase, viral infections, injection-site reactions, pruritis[119]

Abbreviations: AD, atopic dermatitis; CSU, chronic spontaneous urticaria; EoE, eosinophilic esophagitis; ICS, inhaled corticosteroid; INCS, intranasal corticosteroid; IV, intravenous; OCS, oral corticosteroid; PN, prurigo nodularis; SC, subcutaneous.

Omalizumab (anti-immunoglobulin E)

Omalizumab is a recombinant humanized IgG1 monoclonal anti-IgE antibody approved for moderate to severe allergic asthma.[3,33–35] In 2003, omalizumab became the first biological agent to be approved for asthma in the United States.[3,34] This medication binds to circulating free IgE, thereby forming inert IgE-anti-IgE complexes. Omalizumab downregulates high-affinity IgE receptors on pro-inflammatory cells and inhibits release of inflammatory mediators from these cell types.[3,33,34] Randomized controlled trials (RCTs) have shown that omalizumab reduces asthma exacerbations, symptoms, lost work or school days, health care utilization, and asthma medication use. The drug increases asthma control, lung function, and quality of life (QOL).[17,34,35] These benefits were observed at 1 year, and emerging evidence suggests effectiveness persists for up to 4 years.[34,35]

Interleukin-5

Eosinophils play a central and well-described role in asthma.[36] Elevated eosinophil counts are associated with asthma severity and exacerbations.[36] IL-5 is a cytokine that contributes to eosinophil development and maturation in the bone marrow and blood precursors.[36] Expression of IL-5 receptors is upregulated on eosinophils in patients with asthma, resulting in increased activation and release of pro-inflammatory mediators, leukotrienes, and histamine, and subsequent airway hyperresponsiveness.[36]

Early trials investigating anti-IL-5 therapies in asthma showed reduction of blood and sputum eosinophils but limited improvement in lung function.[36–38] These studies were conducted in patients with severe asthma; however, patients were not selected based on peripheral eosinophilia.[36] More recent trials accounted for asthma phenotype and revealed anti-IL-5 therapy efficacy in eosinophilic asthma.[36–40] Three anti-IL-5 therapies have been FDA-approved as asthma maintenance medications: mepolizumab, reslizumab, and benralizumab.

Mepolizumab (anti-interleukin-5)

Mepolizumab is an anti-IL-5 humanized mAb that targets the IL-5 ligand and is used for severe refractory eosinophilic asthma in adult patients.[41,42] Mepolizumab reduces differentiation, recruitment, activation, and survival of eosinophils, selectively inhibiting eosinophilic airway inflammation.[36,41,43] Three major trials evaluating the efficacy of mepolizumab were completed: Dose Ranging Efficacy and Safety with Mepolizumab (DREAM) trial, Mepolizumab as Adjunctive Therapy in Patients with Severe Asthma trial, and Steroid Reduction with Mepolizumab Study.[44–46] These trials showed a clinically significant decrease in asthma exacerbations and lower blood and sputum eosinophil counts in patients exposed to mepolizumab compared with placebo.[36,44–47] In the DREAM trial, mepolizumab was well-tolerated for 12 months and demonstrated a significant reduction in the number of asthma exacerbations.[44] The COSMOS trial demonstrated a sustained clinical response after the initial 12-month study periods, suggesting longer term efficacy; however, additional studies are needed to confirm this finding.[36,48]

Reslizumab (anti-interleukin-5)

Reslizumab is an anti-IL-5 humanized mAb that targets the IL-5 ligand and is approved for use in severe asthma with an eosinophilic phenotype.[36,41,49] Similar to mepolizumab, reslizumab neutralizes circulating IL-5 by inhibiting IL-5-eosinophil binding.[39,43,50] Two phase III RCTs showed significant improvements in forced expiratory volume in one second (FEV$_1$), Asthma Quality of Life Questionnaire, Asthma Control Questionnaire-7 (ACQ-7), Asthma Symptom Utility Index scores, and blood eosinophil levels in patients with asthma and eosinophil levels $\geq$ 400 cells/μL.[36,43,49,51] Additional studies confirmed the improvement of lung function in asthmatic patients with baseline eosinophilia and further revealed these changes occurred at 4 and 16 weeks of treatment with reslizumab.[43,52,53] However, following discontinuation of the medication, baseline blood eosinophilia returned.[43] Studies demonstrate that reslizumab is well-tolerated, however, safety data beyond 52 weeks have not been obtained; therefore, the long-term safety profile remains unknown.[36,39,49] This medication is the only biologic for asthma that is administered via intravenous route.

Benralizumab (anti-interleukin-5 receptor)

Benralizumab is an anti-IL-5 humanized mAb that targets the IL-5 receptor α and is used for severe uncontrolled asthma with peripheral blood eosinophilia in adult patients.[41,54] The IL-5 receptor has two subunits: the α subunit is specific for IL-5 and the β subunit has a role in cell signaling.[54] Benralizumab inhibits signaling via the α receptor expressed on eosinophils and basophils, which prevents downstream signaling cascades, inhibits eosinophil proliferation, and causes apoptotic destruction of eosinophils and basophils.[54]

Early preclinical and phase I studies investigating the efficacy of benralizumab in asthma demonstrated a significant reduction in sputum and blood eosinophil levels.[43,55,56] This prompted additional work testing various doses of benralizumab in patients with asthma and found decreased exacerbations and hospitalization rates.[43,57,58] Three major phase IIIa RCTs, CALIMA, SIROCCO, and ZONDA, revealed that patients with eosinophilic asthma treated with benralizumab had improved lung function, decreased exacerbations, reduced requirements for oral corticosteroids (OCS), and improved QOL.[36,43,54,59–62] The greatest effects were observed in individuals with a history of $\geq$ 3 exacerbations and peripheral eosinophil count $\geq$ 300 cells/μL.[36] Additional benefits of benralizumab use include less frequent dosing and the potential to decrease asthma exacerbations despite blood eosinophil count.[54]

Interleukin-4 and interleukin-13

IL-4 and IL-13 are increased in the airways, serum, and sputum in patients with allergic asthma.[41,63] These cytokines are secreted by CD4$^+$ Th2 cells, type 2 innate lymphoid cells, basophils, and eosinophils and are responsible for Ig class switching from IgM to IgE.[41,63] IL-4 and IL-13 activate a heterodimeric receptor complex expressed on airway and inflammatory cell types to stimulate downstream Th2 cell activation target genes, IgE production, mast cell growth, mucous metaplasia, and bronchial remodeling.[63] As a result, patients have increased airway smooth muscle contraction, bronchial hyperresponsiveness, recruitment of airway eosinophils, and mucus production.[63]

Dupilumab (anti-interleukin-4α receptor)

Dupilumab is a human mAb targeting the α subunit of the IL-4 receptor and the IL-4 and IL-13 signal transduction pathways for individuals with persistent, moderate to severe asthma.[41,63]

RCTs demonstrated that dupilumab use decreases exacerbations, improves FEV_1, improves asthma control score (ACS), and decreases OCS use.[18,19,43,63–65] Biomarkers associated with Th2 inflammation such as FE_{NO}, IgE, and eotaxin-2 were significantly decreased with dupilumab use.[63] Similar benefits were found in pediatric patients.[43,66] These findings were observed independent of circulating eosinophil count, demonstrating appropriate efficacy of dupilumab in patients with severe asthma and OCS-dependent asthma.[18,43] Efficacy is maintained for up to 1 year in patients with uncontrolled asthma and one study suggested additional long-term, sustained improvements in efficacy for up to 148 weeks.[67] Future studies are needed to confirm these findings.[67]

Thymic stromal lymphopoietin

Thymic stromal lymphopoietin (TSLP) is a cytokine produced by epithelial cells, keratinocytes, stromal cells, and allergen-activated basophils during exposure to inhaled environmental allergens and pollutants.[68–71] TSLP induces multiple cell lineages to proliferate, differentiate, and produce pro-inflammatory cytokines, contributing to Th2 and non-Th2 inflammation.[68,69,71] In addition, TSLP may increase collagen produced by fibroblasts and airway smooth muscle proliferation, resulting in airway remodeling.[70] In patients with asthma, increased TSLP expression correlates with impaired lung function, severe disease, and poor response to corticosteroid therapy.[68,69,71]

Tezepelumab (anti-thymic stromal lymphopoietin)

Tezepelumab is a human IgG2 monoclonal anti-TSLP antibody approved for use in patients with severe asthma.[68,70,71] This medication inhibits TSLP preventing binding to its receptor complex and inhibits Th2 cytokines.[68] Tezepelumab is the first biologic agent intended for use in severe asthma without specific criteria such as blood eosinophil counts, biomarkers, and FE_{NO}, or phenotypes.[68] RCTs have shown that tezepelumab improves FEV_1, exacerbations, FE_{NO} levels, and eosinophil count in patients with various asthma phenotypes.[68,70,71] These studies evaluated outcomes through 52 weeks and longer term study would be beneficial.[68]

Selection, Monitoring, and Continuation of Asthma Medications

Selection and initiation of biologic agents depends on a multitude of factors. First, determining suitability for treatment with a biologic agent depends on the eligibility criteria. Number of exacerbations, OCS use, biomarker levels (eosinophil count, FE_{NO}, serum total IgE, allergen-specific IgE), symptoms, FEV_1, and QOL are the key factors considered.[72] It is important to evaluate patients for specific asthma phenotypes and biomarkers to determine the most appropriate and targeted biologic agent. Other relevant considerations include frequency of dosing schedule, route of administration, monitoring by health care personnel during administration, age at asthma onset, coexisting conditions, insurance coverage, out-of-pocket cost, and patient preference.[72,73] Determining when to initiate a biologic medication and selecting the most appropriate agent can be challenging. To date, there remain no data from head-to-head RCTs comparing the approved biologic medications in severe asthma.[72,74,75]

Following initiation, ongoing monitoring remains important. Current guidelines state that patient response to biologic treatment should be monitored after 3 to 4 months of medication initiation and every 3 to 6 months thereafter.[76,77] Patients should be asked about exacerbations, symptoms, QOL, adherence, satisfaction, and safety issues.[72,76,77] Additional workup may include tracking corticosteroid dose reductions, use of health care services, improvements in lung function, and effect on coexisting conditions.[72,78,79] If the patient has a good response to biologic therapy, providers may consider first gradually decreasing OCS therapy, followed by decreasing inhaled treatments after 3 to 6 months.[76,77,80] At a minimum, medium-dose inhaled treatments should be continued.[76,77,80] There are limited studies evaluating withdrawal of biologic therapy; current recommendations state stopping a biologic should not be considered until at least 12 months of treatment, and at this time, the patient must have well-controlled asthma on medium-dose inhaled corticosteroid (ICS) therapy without exposure to allergic triggers.[76,77]

If the patient has a poor response to a biologic agent, it is critical to review factors contributing to symptoms, consider additional clinical testing, and discuss alternative treatment options.[76,77] If considering an alternative biologic agent, the patient should be reevaluated for asthma phenotype and specific biomarkers.[72,76,77] Currently, coadministration of multiple biologic agents is not recommended due to the lack of evidence and high cost.[72]

Biological Management of Nasal Polyps

Similar to asthma, biologic agents serve as an adjunctive treatment for CRSwNP and target type 2 inflammation.[81] There are three biologic medications that are FDA-approved for CRSwNP: omalizumab, dupilumab, and mepolizumab. Here, we outline the mechanism, clinical trials, and efficacy of these agents in CRSwNP.

Omalizumab (anti-immunoglobulin E)

IgE-mediated inflammation plays a significant role in CRSwNP and contributes to symptomatology.[31,32] High concentrations of IgE are found in NPs, in addition to IgA, IgG, B cells, and plasma cells.[82] Omalizumab was approved in 2020 for use in CRSwNP and serves to modulate IgE in type 2 inflammation.[82] POLYP 1 and POLYP 2 were two multicenter RCTs that evaluated the efficacy and safety of omalizumab for the management of CRSwNP refractory to intranasal corticosteroids.[83] These studies found that omalizumab decreased endoscopic NP scores, nasal congestion scores, and the 22-item Sinonasal Outcome Test (SNOT-22) scores after 24 weeks.[83]

Mepolizumab (anti-interleukin-5)

Eosinophils are known to accumulate in the nasal mucosa of patients with CRSwNP.[81] IL-5 contributes to prolonged survival, differentiation, and accumulation of eosinophils in nasal mucosa, and higher levels of IL-5 have been associated with worse NPs.[81] Mepolizumab is an anti-IL-5 biologic therapy approved for use in CRSwNPs in 2021.[81] The SYNAPSE trial was a multicenter RCT that investigated the effect of mepolizumab on CRSwNP in patients who previously underwent sinus surgery and were refractory to ongoing treatments.[84] This study demonstrated that mepolizumab resulted in improved endoscopic NP scores and decreased nasal obstruction after 52 weeks of treatment.[84]

Dupilumab (anti-interleukin-4α receptor)

IL-4 and IL-13 are upregulated and contribute to a pro-inflammatory environment in CRSwNP.[85] In NPs, these cytokines activate epithelial cells to enhance upper airway remodeling, resulting in hyperplasia, excess mucus secretion, and type III collagen production.[85] Dupilumab is an anti-IL-4/IL-13 biologic agent that attenuates sinonasal inflammation and was approved for use in CRSwNP in 2017.[85] The LIBERTY NP SINUS-24 and LIBERTY NP SINUS-52 were two multicenter RCTs that evaluated the effects of dupilumab for CRSwNP refractory to medical or surgical treatments after 24 and 52 weeks, respectively.[86] These two trials found that dupilumab improved NP scores, nasal congestion or obstruction scores, SNOT-22 scores, Lund-Mackay scores, and sinonasal QOL.[86,87]

Candidacy and Selection of Biologic Therapies for Nasal Polyps

The decision on when to start a biological therapy is nuanced and many factors must be considered before medication initiation. One study compared a prospective cohort of individuals with CRSwNP who underwent functional endoscopic sinus surgery (FESS) with patients included in phase III biologic trials for omalizumab, dupilumab, and mepolizumab.[88] This study found that FESS resulted in greater reduction of polyp size compared with all three biologics. In addition, FESS and dupilumab resulted in similar improvements in the SNOT-22 scores. However, compared with omalizumab,

FESS resulted in better improvement in SNOT-22 scores. Dupilumab and FESS resulted in similar improvement in smell identification at 24 weeks.

Multiple studies have found that FESS is more cost-effective than biologic medications; thus, current guidelines generally advocate starting with FESS, rather than biologics, in individuals who have failed other medical therapies.[88–91] However, there are exceptions to this, including patients with contraindications to undergoing surgery and those who would benefit from a biologic for poorly controlled comorbid asthma. In 2023, the European Position paper on Rhinosinusitis and Nasal Polyps (EPOS) and European Forum for Research and Education in Allergy and Airway Diseases (EUFOREA) published an update on biologics for CRSwNP.[26] This document provides specific indications for when to consider biologic therapy (**Fig. 1**). All patients must have bilateral NPs and either have had prior FESS or be unfit to undergo surgery. In addition, patients must meet at least three of the criteria listed: evidence of type 2 inflammation, need for frequent systemic steroids or have a contraindication to systemic steroids, significantly impaired QOL, significant loss of smell, or have a diagnosis of comorbid asthma.

Once a patient is determined to be a candidate for biologic therapy, providers select the specific biologic to be used. There have been no head-to-head RCTs directly comparing the three biologics that are FDA-approved for CRSwNP. However, indirect treatment comparisons have found dupilumab to be most efficacious in treating CRSwNP.[92,93] One study compared two RCTs on dupilumab and two RCTs on omalizumab for CRSwNP.[92] Here, patients on dupilumab had significantly greater improvements in outcome measures from baseline to 24 weeks of treatment. Specifically, patients on dupilumab had improved NP scores, nasal congestion, olfactory function, and total symptom scores.[92] Another study compared seven RCTs that included dupilumab, mepolizumab, omalizumab, and benralizumab (FDA-approved for asthma, but not CRSwNP).[93] This study found that dupilumab was more efficacious in decreasing NP scores and nasal congestion, compared with the other three biologics after 24 weeks of treatment and at the end of follow-up (>48 weeks). In addition, there were no significant differences in rates of adverse events following treatment with these four biologics.[93]

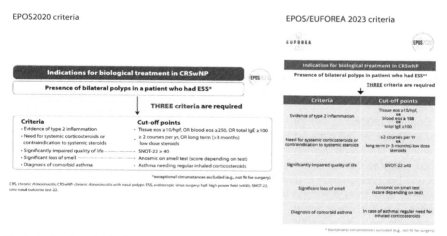

EPOS2020 criteria

EPOS/EUFOREA 2023 criteria

Fig. 1. Indications for biological treatment in chronic rhinosinusitis with nasal polyposis. All candidates must have bilateral nasal polyps and prior endoscopic sinus surgery (ESS). There are exceptional circumstances where no prior ESS is required (i.e. not fit for surgery). *From* Fokkense WJ, et al. EPOS/EUFOREA update on indication and evaluation of Biologics in Chronic Rhinosinusitis with Nasal Polyps 2023. Rhinology, 2023. 61(3): p. 194-202.

Opportunities to Enhance Care with Biologic Treatments

Challenges remain with the use of biologic agents in the treatment of asthma and CRSwNP. Biologic medications are expensive, and cost remains a significant barrier to use of these drugs.[94–96] Data offered by pharmaceutical manufacturers state that wholesale cost for one unit of these biologic agents ranges from $879 to more than $4750, not including additional fees charged by health care providers for medication administration or appointments.[94] Biologic agents are not yet cost-effective, and one group argued that the cost of these medications would need to be reduced by 62% to 80% to be cost-effective in comparison to current asthma medications.[94] In addition, one study revealed that insurance approval further complicates this process; prior authorization for biologic agents may be slow and patients with asthma are at risk for exacerbations and increased need for OCS during this time.[97]

Clinically, ongoing challenges include outcomes, administration, and medication candidacy. Antidrug antibodies develop in nonhuman species treated with biologic agents, which raises concern for the development of these antibodies in humans.[98] Research to better understand the mechanism of antidrug antibodies and other neutralizing molecules are underway.[98,99] Route and ease of administration is another concern, particularly for intravenous reslizumab; however, subcutaneous studies are ongoing.[100] Challenges in measuring efficacy of biologic agents also remain a concern. The development of improved clinical and serum markers, outcome measures (ie, SNOT-22), and standardized follow-up care will allow for better understanding of patient progress. Last, patient candidacy remains a challenge for specific disease populations, such as patients with cystic fibrosis and NPs. Future research endeavors should investigate whether biologics can be used in these populations.[101]

FUTURE DIRECTIONS FOR BIOLOGIC TREATMENTS

Despite significant advancements in these novel therapies, opportunities remain to better incorporate biologic agents into clinical care. First, establishing reliable biomarkers would help guide treatment and monitoring of biologic therapies.[72] Evaluating antidrug antibodies would help reveal potential for decreased drug efficacy.[72] Further understanding length of treatment time, effect of biologics on the course of disease, change in endotypes, and whether these medications might ameliorate disease are needed.[72] Expanding clinical trials to evaluate specific populations such as children and adolescents may lead to additional indications for biologic medications.[72,102,103] Head-to-head comparison trials are needed to compare the effectiveness of each biologic agent and to improve our ability to target the correct cohort of patients.[72,74,75]

Ongoing studies to further investigate approved drugs are underway. Two future phase IV studies are planned to provide additional safety and efficacy data for mepolizumab.[36] The Mepolizumab Pregnancy Exposure Study is a post-marketing surveillance study to further understand mepolizumab safety in pregnant patients.[36] The second upcoming study is a multinational observational study to evaluate the effectiveness and to understand mepolizumab's use in clinical practice.[36] Additional work to develop novel anti-IL-13 mAbs for patients with moderate to severe uncontrolled asthma and severe OCS-dependent asthma is also underway; however, multiple phase III trials for tralokinumab and lebrikizumab showed no clinically significant improvements in FEV_1 or exacerbations.[41,43]

Current biologic agents being studied target biomarkers and cytokines not previously investigated. Fevipiprant is a nonsteroidal oral prostaglandin D2 receptor antagonist for patients with asthma.[104] Studies demonstrated that fevipiprant reduces bronchial wall inflammation, increasing FEV_1, decreased ACQ scores, and decreased exacerbations.[104] IL-25 and IL-33 also have potential in the treatment of asthma.[105] No biologic medications targeting IL-25 are currently under investigation; however, two anti-IL-33 biologic agents are being studied including itepekimab and etokimab.[43,105] Other targets currently being studied include CRTH2 and STAT5/6 Src homology 2 domains.[105]

Ongoing work to evaluate benralizumab and reslizumab for CRSwNP is underway.[106] The recent phase III OSTRO study found that NP score, NP blockage score, and clinical symptoms such as olfactory dysfunction significantly improved after 40 weeks of treatment with benralizumab.[106] Enhanced response was observed in subgroups with comorbid asthma and increased peripheral eosinophil counts.[106] Studies evaluating reslizumab remain limited at this time; however, recent work suggests a potential role as an adjunctive therapy in patients with CRSwNP.[107] A post hoc analysis of the phase III NAVIGATOR study found that individuals with severe asthma and CRSwNP who were on tezepelumab had improvements in their SNOT-22 scores over 52 weeks of treatment.[108] The WAYPOINT phase III trial is currently ongoing to evaluate the efficacy and safety of tezepelumab for CRSwNP.[109]

Potential targets to treat CRS include the Th1, Th2, and Th17 inflammatory pathways may be the focus of biologic agent development.[110] IFN-gamma inducible protein 10 (CXCL10) plays a role in inflammation persistence and studies have demonstrated increased expression levels of CXCL10 in nasal fibroblasts of patients with type 2 CRS.[110,111] In addition, tumor necrosis factor receptor OX40 expression is increased in dendritic cells of NPs.[110,112]

SUMMARY

Accurate endotyping in asthma and CRS is emerging to guide targeted treatments with biologic agents. Recent RCTs target specific endotypes and use strict eligibility criteria.[36] Research efforts are focused on improving our understanding of Th2-mediated inflammation and other inflammatory pathways, with the goal of developing novel targets, drugs, and biomarkers. This work will allow for individualized treatment of patients with asthma and CRSwNP. Future work should explore biologic agent accessibility, cost, and applicability in other related disease processes.

CLINICS CARE POINTS

- Number of asthma exacerbations, oral corticosteroids use, symptoms, lung function, and quality of life (QOL) are the key factors considered in the workup before initiation of biologic treatment in asthma.

- Bilateral nasal polyps, prior functional endoscopic sinus surgery or surgical eligibility, presence of type 2 inflammation, systemic steroid use, QOL, loss of smell, and comorbid asthma are considered before initiation of biologic treatment in chronic rhinosinusitis.

- Patient preferences play an important role in selecting the appropriate biologic agent including dosing frequency, route of administration, insurance, and out-of-pocket costs.

- Patients treated with biologic agents should be evaluated after 3 to 4 months of medication initiation and every 3 to 6 months thereafter for exacerbations, symptoms, adherence, satisfaction, and safety issues.

- Other asthma medications may be slowly discontinued once a biologic agent has been deemed efficacious and safe; however, patients should continue a medium-dose inhaled corticosteroid regardless of biologic agent efficacy.

DISCLOSURES

H.K. Mandl: none. J.E. Miller: none. D.M. Beswick: In the last 36 months, unrelated to this work, D.M. Beswick has received grant support from CF Foundation, the International Society of Inflammation and Allergy of the Nose, and the Sue Ann and John L. Weinberg Foundation, honoraria, and consulting fees from Amgen, on medicolegal cases and at Garner Health (equity).

REFERENCES

1. Olin JT, Wechsler ME. Asthma: pathogenesis and novel drugs for treatment. BMJ 2014;349:g5517.
2. Kuruvilla ME, Lee FE, Lee GB. Understanding Asthma Phenotypes, Endotypes, and Mechanisms of Disease. Clin Rev Allergy Immunol 2019;56(2):219–33.
3. Jin HJ. Biological treatments for severe asthma. Yeungnam Univ J Med 2020; 37(4):262–8.
4. Blackwell DL, Lucas JW, Clarke TC. Summary health statistics for U.S. adults: national health interview survey, 2012. Vital Health Stat 2014;10(260):1–161.
5. Bhattacharyya N, Gilani S. Prevalence of Potential Adult Chronic Rhinosinusitis Symptoms in the United States. Otolaryngol Head Neck Surg 2018;159(3): 522–5.
6. Soler ZM, Mace JC, Litvack JR, et al. Chronic rhinosinusitis, race, and ethnicity. Am J Rhinol Allergy 2012;26(2):110–6.
7. Hirsch AG, Stewart WF, Sundaresan AS, et al. Nasal and sinus symptoms and chronic rhinosinusitis in a population-based sample. Allergy 2017;72(2):274–81.
8. DeConde AS, Soler ZM. Chronic rhinosinusitis: Epidemiology and burden of disease. Am J Rhinol Allergy 2016;30(2):134–9.
9. Shi JB, Fu QL, Zhang H, et al. Epidemiology of chronic rhinosinusitis: results from a cross-sectional survey in seven Chinese cities. Allergy 2015;70(5):533–9.
10. Orlandi RR, Kingdom TT, Smith TL, et al. International consensus statement on allergy and rhinology: rhinosinusitis 2021. Int Forum Allergy Rhinol 2021;11(3): 213–739.
11. Tomassen P, Vandeplas G, Van Zele T, et al. Inflammatory endotypes of chronic rhinosinusitis based on cluster analysis of biomarkers. J Allergy Clin Immunol 2016;137(5):1449–56.e4.
12. Klossek JM, Neukirch F, Pribil C, et al. Prevalence of nasal polyposis in France: a cross-sectional, case-control study. Allergy 2005;60(2):233–7.
13. Hedman J, Kaprio J, Poussa T, et al. Prevalence of asthma, aspirin intolerance, nasal polyposis and chronic obstructive pulmonary disease in a population-based study. Int J Epidemiol 1999;28(4):717–22.
14. Johansson L, Akerlund A, Holmberg K, et al. Prevalence of nasal polyps in adults: the Skövde population-based study. Ann Otol Rhinol Laryngol 2003; 112(7):625–9.
15. Ahn JC, Kim JW, Lee CH, et al. Prevalence and Risk Factors of Chronic Rhinosinusitus, Allergic Rhinitis, and Nasal Septal Deviation: Results of the Korean National Health and Nutrition Survey 2008-2012. JAMA Otolaryngol Head Neck Surg 2016;142(2):162–7.
16. Anderson GP. Endotyping asthma: new insights into key pathogenic mechanisms in a complex, heterogeneous disease. Lancet 2008;372(9643):1107–19.
17. Hamilton D, Lehman H. Asthma Phenotypes as a Guide for Current and Future Biologic Therapies. Clin Rev Allergy Immunol 2020;59(2):160–74.

18. Castro M, Corren J, Pavord ID, et al. Dupilumab Efficacy and Safety in Moderate-to-Severe Uncontrolled Asthma. N Engl J Med 2018;378(26): 2486–96.

19. Rabe KF, Nair P, Brusselle G, et al. Efficacy and Safety of Dupilumab in Glucocorticoid-Dependent Severe Asthma. N Engl J Med 2018;378(26): 2475–85.

20. Akdis CA, Bachert C, Cingi C, et al. Endotypes and phenotypes of chronic rhinosinusitis: a PRACTALL document of the European Academy of Allergy and Clinical Immunology and the American Academy of Allergy, Asthma & Immunology. J Allergy Clin Immunol 2013;131(6):1479–90.

21. Turner JH, Chandra RK, Li P, et al. Identification of clinically relevant chronic rhinosinusitis endotypes using cluster analysis of mucus cytokines. J Allergy Clin Immunol 2018;141(5):1895–7.e7.

22. Divekar R, Rank M, Squillace D, et al. Unsupervised network mapping of commercially available immunoassay yields three distinct chronic rhinosinusitis endotypes. Int Forum Allergy Rhinol 2017;7(4):373–9.

23. Liao B, Liu JX, Li ZY, et al. Multidimensional endotypes of chronic rhinosinusitis and their association with treatment outcomes. Allergy 2018;73(7):1459–69.

24. Hoggard M, Waldvogel-Thurlow S, Zoing M, et al. Inflammatory Endotypes and Microbial Associations in Chronic Rhinosinusitis. Front Immunol 2018;9:2065.

25. Ahern S, Cervin A. Inflammation and Endotyping in Chronic Rhinosinusitis-A Paradigm Shift. Medicina (Kaunas) 2019;55(4):95.

26. Fokkens WJ, Viskens AS, Backer V, et al. EPOS/EUFOREA update on indication and evaluation of Biologics in Chronic Rhinosinusitis with Nasal Polyps 2023. Rhinology 2023;61(3):194–202.

27. Krouse JH, Brown RW, Fineman SM, et al. Asthma and the unified airway. Otolaryngol Head Neck Surg 2007;136(5 Suppl):S75–106.

28. Fokkens W, Reitsma S. Unified Airway Disease: A Contemporary Review and Introduction. Otolaryngol Clin North Am 2023;56(1):1–10.

29. Ahmad JG, Marino MJ, Luong AU. Unified Airway Disease: Future Directions. Otolaryngol Clin North Am 2023;56(1):181–95.

30. Chong LY, Piromchai P, Sharp S, et al. Biologics for chronic rhinosinusitis. Cochrane Database Syst Rev 2021;3(3):Cd013513.

31. Froidure A, Mouthuy J, Durham SR, et al. Asthma phenotypes and IgE responses. Eur Respir J 2016;47(1):304–19.

32. Gould HJ, Sutton BJ. IgE in allergy and asthma today. Nat Rev Immunol 2008; 8(3):205–17.

33. Strunk RC, Bloomberg GR. Omalizumab for asthma. N Engl J Med 2006; 354(25):2689–95.

34. MacDonald KM, Kavati A, Ortiz B, et al. Short- and long-term real-world effectiveness of omalizumab in severe allergic asthma: systematic review of 42 studies published 2008-2018. Expert Rev Clin Immunol 2019;15(5):553–69.

35. Bousquet J, Humbert M, Gibson PG, et al. Real-World Effectiveness of Omalizumab in Severe Allergic Asthma: A Meta-Analysis of Observational Studies. J Allergy Clin Immunol Pract 2021;9(7):2702–14.

36. Leung E, Al Efraij K, FitzGerald JM. The safety of mepolizumab for the treatment of asthma. Expert Opin Drug Saf 2017;16(3):397–404.

37. Leckie MJ, ten Brinke A, Khan J, et al. Effects of an interleukin-5 blocking monoclonal antibody on eosinophils, airway hyper-responsiveness, and the late asthmatic response. Lancet 2000;356(9248):2144–8.

38. Flood-Page P, Swenson C, Faiferman I, et al. A study to evaluate safety and efficacy of mepolizumab in patients with moderate persistent asthma. Am J Respir Crit Care Med 2007;176(11):1062–71.
39. Castro M, Mathur S, Hargreave F, et al. Reslizumab for poorly controlled, eosinophilic asthma: a randomized, placebo-controlled study. Am J Respir Crit Care Med 2011;184(10):1125–32.
40. Hargreave FE, Nair P. Point: Is Measuring Sputum Eosinophils Useful Management Severe Asthma? Yes. Chest 2011;139(6):1270–3.
41. Santini G, Mores N, Malerba M, et al. Dupilumab for the treatment of asthma. Expert Opin Investig Drugs 2017;26(3):357–66.
42. Skloot GS. Asthma phenotypes and endotypes: a personalized approach to treatment. Curr Opin Pulm Med 2016;22(1):3–9.
43. Ramírez-Jiménez F, Pavón-Romero GF, Velásquez-Rodríguez JM, et al. Biologic Therapies for Asthma and Allergic Disease: Past, Present, and Future. Pharmaceuticals (Basel) 2023;16(2):270.
44. Pavord ID, Korn S, Howarth P, et al. Mepolizumab for severe eosinophilic asthma (DREAM): a multicentre, double-blind, placebo-controlled trial. Lancet 2012;380(9842):651–9.
45. Ortega HG, Liu MC, Pavord ID, et al. Mepolizumab treatment in patients with severe eosinophilic asthma. N Engl J Med 2014;371(13):1198–207.
46. Bel EH, Wenzel SE, Thompson PJ, et al. Oral glucocorticoid-sparing effect of mepolizumab in eosinophilic asthma. N Engl J Med 2014;371(13):1189–97.
47. Haldar P, Brightling CE, Hargadon B, et al. Mepolizumab and exacerbations of refractory eosinophilic asthma. N Engl J Med 2009;360(10):973–84.
48. Lugogo N, Domingo C, Chanez P, et al. Long-term Efficacy and Safety of Mepolizumab in Patients With Severe Eosinophilic Asthma: A Multi-center, Open-label, Phase IIIb Study. Clin Ther 2016;38(9):2058–70.e1.
49. Castro M, Zangrilli J, Wechsler ME, et al. Reslizumab for inadequately controlled asthma with elevated blood eosinophil counts: results from two multicentre, parallel, double-blind, randomised, placebo-controlled, phase 3 trials. Lancet Respir Med 2015;3(5):355–66.
50. Khatri S, Moore W, Gibson PG, et al. Assessment of the long-term safety of mepolizumab and durability of clinical response in patients with severe eosinophilic asthma. J Allergy Clin Immunol 2019;143(5):1742–51.e7.
51. Bjermer L, Lemiere C, Maspero J, et al. Reslizumab for Inadequately Controlled Asthma With Elevated Blood Eosinophil Levels: A Randomized Phase 3 Study. Chest 2016;150(4):789–98.
52. Corren J, Weinstein S, Janka L, et al. Phase 3 Study of Reslizumab in Patients With Poorly Controlled Asthma: Effects Across a Broad Range of Eosinophil Counts. Chest 2016;150(4):799–810.
53. Murphy K, Jacobs J, Bjermer L, et al. Long-term Safety and Efficacy of Reslizumab in Patients with Eosinophilic Asthma. J Allergy Clin Immunol Pract 2017;5(6):1572–81.e3.
54. Saco TV, Pepper AN, Lockey RF. Benralizumab for the treatment of asthma. Expert Rev Clin Immunol 2017;13(5):405–13.
55. Busse WW, Katial R, Gossage D, et al. Safety profile, pharmacokinetics, and biologic activity of MEDI-563, an anti-IL-5 receptor alpha antibody, in a phase I study of subjects with mild asthma. J Allergy Clin Immunol 2010;125(6):1237–44.e2.

56. Laviolette M, Gossage DL, Gauvreau G, et al. Effects of benralizumab on airway eosinophils in asthmatic patients with sputum eosinophilia. J Allergy Clin Immunol 2013;132(5):1086–96.e5.
57. Castro M, Wenzel SE, Bleecker ER, et al. Benralizumab, an anti-interleukin 5 receptor α monoclonal antibody, versus placebo for uncontrolled eosinophilic asthma: a phase 2b randomised dose-ranging study. Lancet Respir Med 2014;2(11):879–90.
58. Nowak RM, Parker JM, Silverman RA, et al. A randomized trial of benralizumab, an antiinterleukin 5 receptor α monoclonal antibody, after acute asthma. Am J Emerg Med 2015;33(1):14–20.
59. FitzGerald JM, Bleecker ER, Nair P, et al. Benralizumab, an anti-interleukin-5 receptor α monoclonal antibody, as add-on treatment for patients with severe, uncontrolled, eosinophilic asthma (CALIMA): a randomised, double-blind, placebo-controlled phase 3 trial. Lancet 2016;388(10056):2128–41.
60. Bleecker ER, FitzGerald JM, Chanez P, et al. Efficacy and safety of benralizumab for patients with severe asthma uncontrolled with high-dosage inhaled corticosteroids and long-acting β(2)-agonists (SIROCCO): a randomised, multicentre, placebo-controlled phase 3 trial. Lancet 2016;388(10056):2115–27.
61. Maselli DJ, Rogers L, Peters JI. Benralizumab, an add-on treatment for severe eosinophilic asthma: evaluation of exacerbations, emergency department visits, lung function, and oral corticosteroid use. Ther Clin Risk Manag 2018;14: 2059–68.
62. Nair P, Wenzel S, Rabe KF, et al. Oral Glucocorticoid-Sparing Effect of Benralizumab in Severe Asthma. N Engl J Med 2017;376(25):2448–58.
63. Vatrella A, Fabozzi I, Calabrese C, et al. Dupilumab: a novel treatment for asthma. J Asthma Allergy 2014;7:123–30.
64. Wenzel S, Ford L, Pearlman D, et al. Dupilumab in persistent asthma with elevated eosinophil levels. N Engl J Med 2013;368(26):2455–66.
65. Wenzel S, Castro M, Corren J, et al. Dupilumab efficacy and safety in adults with uncontrolled persistent asthma despite use of medium-to-high-dose inhaled corticosteroids plus a long-acting β2 agonist: a randomised double-blind placebo-controlled pivotal phase 2b dose-ranging trial. Lancet 2016;388(10039): 31–44.
66. Bacharier LB, Maspero JF, Katelaris CH, et al. Dupilumab in Children with Uncontrolled Moderate-to-Severe Asthma. N Engl J Med 2021;385(24):2230–40.
67. Wechsler ME, Ford LB, Maspero JF, et al. Long-term safety and efficacy of dupilumab in patients with moderate-to-severe asthma (TRAVERSE): an open-label extension study. Lancet Respir Med 2022;10(1):11–25.
68. Zoumot Z, Al Busaidi N, Tashkandi W, et al. Tezepelumab for Patients with Severe Uncontrolled Asthma: A Systematic Review and Meta-Analysis. J Asthma Allergy 2022;15:1665–79.
69. Rochman Y, Leonard WJ. Thymic stromal lymphopoietin: a new cytokine in asthma. Curr Opin Pharmacol 2008;8(3):249–54.
70. Diver S, Khalfaoui L, Emson C, et al. Effect of tezepelumab on airway inflammatory cells, remodelling, and hyperresponsiveness in patients with moderate-to-severe uncontrolled asthma (CASCADE): a double-blind, randomised, placebo-controlled, phase 2 trial. Lancet Respir Med 2021;9(11):1299–312.
71. Corren J, Ambrose CS, Sałapa K, et al. Efficacy of Tezepelumab in Patients with Severe, Uncontrolled Asthma and Perennial Allergy. J Allergy Clin Immunol Pract 2021;9(12):4334–42.e6.

72. Brusselle GG, Koppelman GH. Biologic Therapies for Severe Asthma. N Engl J Med 2022;386(2):157–71.

73. Krings JG, McGregor MC, Bacharier LB, et al. Biologics for Severe Asthma: Treatment-Specific Effects Are Important in Choosing a Specific Agent. J Allergy Clin Immunol Pract 2019;7(5):1379–92.

74. Pilette C, Brightling C, Lacombe D, et al. Urgent need for pragmatic trial platforms in severe asthma. Lancet Respir Med 2018;6(8):581–3.

75. Eger K, Kroes JA, Ten Brinke A, et al. Long-Term Therapy Response to Anti-IL-5 Biologics in Severe Asthma-A Real-Life Evaluation. J Allergy Clin Immunol Pract 2021;9(3):1194–200.

76. Reddel HK, Bacharier LB, Bateman ED, et al. Global Initiative for Asthma Strategy 2021: Executive Summary and Rationale for Key Changes. Am J Respir Crit Care Med 2022;205(1):17–35.

77. Levy ML, Bacharier LB, Bateman E, et al. Key recommendations for primary care from the 2022 Global Initiative for Asthma (GINA) update. NPJ Prim Care Respir Med 2023;33(1):7.

78. Israel E, Reddel HK. Severe and Difficult-to-Treat Asthma in Adults. N Engl J Med 2017;377(10):965–76.

79. Pepper AN, Hanania NA, Humbert M, et al. How to Assess Effectiveness of Biologics for Asthma and What Steps to Take When There Is Not Benefit. J Allergy Clin Immunol Pract 2021;9(3):1081–8.

80. Jeffery MM, Inselman JW, Maddux JT, et al. Asthma Patients Who Stop Asthma Biologics Have a Similar Risk of Asthma Exacerbations as Those Who Continue Asthma Biologics. J Allergy Clin Immunol Pract 2021;9(7):2742–50.e1.

81. Gevaert P, Han JK, Smith SG, et al. The roles of eosinophils and interleukin-5 in the pathophysiology of chronic rhinosinusitis with nasal polyps. Int Forum Allergy Rhinol 2022;12(11):1413–23.

82. Kariyawasam HH, James LK. Chronic Rhinosinusitis with Nasal Polyps: Targeting IgE with Anti-IgE Omalizumab Therapy. Drug Des Devel Ther 2020;14:5483–94.

83. Gevaert P, Omachi TA, Corren J, et al. Efficacy and safety of omalizumab in nasal polyposis: 2 randomized phase 3 trials. J Allergy Clin Immunol 2020;146(3):595–605.

84. Han JK, Bachert C, Fokkens W, et al. Mepolizumab for chronic rhinosinusitis with nasal polyps (SYNAPSE): a randomised, double-blind, placebo-controlled, phase 3 trial. Lancet Respir Med 2021;9(10):1141–53.

85. Kariyawasam HH. Chronic rhinosinusitis with nasal polyps: mechanistic insights from targeting IL-4 and IL-13 via IL-4Rα inhibition with dupilumab. Expert Rev Clin Immunol 2020;16(12):1115–25.

86. Bachert C, Han JK, Desrosiers M, et al. Efficacy and safety of dupilumab in patients with severe chronic rhinosinusitis with nasal polyps (LIBERTY NP SINUS-24 and LIBERTY NP SINUS-52): results from two multicentre, randomised, double-blind, placebo-controlled, parallel-group phase 3 trials. Lancet 2019;394(10209):1638–50.

87. Lee SE, Hopkins C, Mullol J, et al. Dupilumab improves health related quality of life: Results from the phase 3 SINUS studies. Allergy 2022;77(7):2211–21.

88. Miglani A, Soler ZM, Smith TL, et al. A comparative analysis of endoscopic sinus surgery versus biologics for treatment of chronic rhinosinusitis with nasal polyposis. Int Forum Allergy Rhinol 2023;13(2):116–28.

89. van der Lans RJL, Hopkins C, Senior BA, et al. Biologicals and Endoscopic Sinus Surgery for Severe Uncontrolled Chronic Rhinosinusitis With Nasal Polyps: An Economic Perspective. J Allergy Clin Immunol Pract 2022;10(6):1454–61.
90. Rathi VK, Scangas GA, Metson RB, et al. Out-of-pocket costs of biologic treatments for chronic rhinosinusitis with nasal polyposis in the Medicare population. Int Forum Allergy Rhinol 2022;12(10):1295–8.
91. Roland LT, Regenberg A, Luong AU, et al. Biologics for chronic rhinosinusitis with nasal polyps: Economics and ethics. Int Forum Allergy Rhinol 2021; 11(11):1524–8.
92. Peters AT, Han JK, Hellings P, et al. Indirect Treatment Comparison of Biologics in Chronic Rhinosinusitis with Nasal Polyps. J Allergy Clin Immunol Pract 2021; 9(6):2461–71.e5.
93. Cai S, Xu S, Lou H, et al. Comparison of Different Biologics for Treating Chronic Rhinosinusitis With Nasal Polyps: A Network Analysis. J Allergy Clin Immunol Pract 2022;10(7):1876–86.e7.
94. Anderson WC 3rd, Szefler SJ. Cost-effectiveness and comparative effectiveness of biologic therapy for asthma: To biologic or not to biologic? Ann Allergy Asthma Immunol 2019;122(4):367–72.
95. Hardtstock F, Krieger J, Wilke T, et al. Use of Biologic Therapies in the Treatment of Asthma - A Comparative Real World Data Analysis on Healthcare Resource Utilization and Costs Before and After Therapy Initiation. J Asthma Allergy 2022;15:407–18.
96. Faverio P, Ronco R, Monzio Compagnoni M, et al. Effectiveness and economic impact of Dupilumab in asthma: a population-based cohort study. Respir Res 2023;24(1):70.
97. Dudiak GJ, Popyack J, Grimm C, et al. Prior authorization delays biologic initiation and is associated with a risk of asthma exacerbations. Allergy Asthma Proc 2021;42(1):65–71.
98. Andrews L, Ralston S, Blomme E, et al. A snapshot of biologic drug development: Challenges and opportunities. Hum Exp Toxicol 2015;34(12):1279–85.
99. Joseph A, Munroe K, Housman M, et al. Immune tolerance induction to enzyme-replacement therapy by co-administration of short-term, low-dose methotrexate in a murine Pompe disease model. Clin Exp Immunol 2008;152(1):138–46.
100. Máspero J. Reslizumab in the treatment of inadequately controlled asthma in adults and adolescents with elevated blood eosinophils: clinical trial evidence and future prospects. Ther Adv Respir Dis 2017;11(8):311–25.
101. Moni SS, Al Basheer A. Molecular targets for cystic fibrosis and therapeutic potential of monoclonal antibodies. Saudi Pharm J 2022;30(12):1736–47.
102. Middleton PG, Gade EJ, Aguilera C, et al. ERS/TSANZ Task Force Statement on the management of reproduction and pregnancy in women with airways diseases. Eur Respir J 2020;55(2):1901208.
103. Pfaller B, José Yepes-Nuñez J, Agache I, et al. Biologicals in atopic disease in pregnancy: An EAACI position paper. Allergy 2021;76(1):71–89.
104. Jahangir A, Sattar SBA, Rafay Khan Niazi M, et al. Efficacy and Safety of Fevipiprant in Asthma: A Review and Meta-Analysis. Cureus 2022;14(5):e24641.
105. Calhoun WJ, Chupp GL. The new era of add-on asthma treatments: where do we stand? Allergy Asthma Clin Immunol 2022;18(1):42.
106. Bachert C, Han JK, Desrosiers MY, et al. Efficacy and safety of benralizumab in chronic rhinosinusitis with nasal polyps: A randomized, placebo-controlled trial. J Allergy Clin Immunol 2022;149(4):1309–17.e12.

107. Kuruvilla ME, Levy J. Efficacy of Reslizumab in Eosinophilic Chronic Sinusitis with Nasal Polyposis. J Allergy Clin Immunol 2018;141(2):AB270.
108. Jacobs J, Hoyte F, Spahn J, et al. Tezepelumab Efficacy By SNOT-22 Score In Patients With Severe, Uncontrolled Asthma And Comorbid Nasal Polyps In NAVIGATOR. J Allergy Clin Immunol 2023;151(2):AB17.
109. Efficacy and Safety of Tezepelumab in Participants With Severe Chronic Rhinosinusitis With Nasal Polyposis (WAYPOINT). 2023 2023-06-23 cited 2023 2023-8-7; Available at: https://clinicaltrials.gov/study/NCT04851964?term=tezepelumab&page=2&rank=11.
110. Tai J, Han M, Kim TH. Therapeutic Strategies of Biologics in Chronic Rhinosinusitis: Current Options and Future Targets. Int J Mol Sci 2022;23(10).
111. Yoshikawa M, Wada K, Yoshimura T, et al. Increased CXCL10 expression in nasal fibroblasts from patients with refractory chronic rhinosinusitis and asthma. Allergol Int 2013;62(4):495–502.
112. Liu T, Li TL, Zhao F, et al. Role of thymic stromal lymphopoietin in the pathogenesis of nasal polyposis. Am J Med Sci 2011;341(1):40–7.
113. Normansell R, Walker S, Milan SJ, et al. Omalizumab for asthma in adults and children. Cochrane Database Syst Rev 2014;1:Cd003559.
114. Busse W, Corren J, Lanier BQ, et al. Omalizumab, anti-IgE recombinant humanized monoclonal antibody, for the treatment of severe allergic asthma. J Allergy Clin Immunol 2001;108(2):184–90.
115. Solèr M, Matz J, Townley R, et al. The anti-IgE antibody omalizumab reduces exacerbations and steroid requirement in allergic asthmatics. Eur Respir J 2001;18(2):254–61.
116. Holgate ST, Chuchalin AG, Hébert J, et al. Efficacy and safety of a recombinant anti-immunoglobulin E antibody (omalizumab) in severe allergic asthma. Clin Exp Allergy 2004;34(4):632–8.
117. Detoraki A, Tremante E, D'Amato M, et al. Mepolizumab improves sino-nasal symptoms and asthma control in severe eosinophilic asthma patients with chronic rhinosinusitis and nasal polyps: a 12-month real-life study. Ther Adv Respir Dis 2021;15. 17534666211009398.
118. Kim J, Naclerio R. Therapeutic Potential of Dupilumab in the Treatment of Chronic Rhinosinusitis with Nasal Polyps: Evidence to Date. Ther Clin Risk Manag 2020;16:31–7.
119. Roy P, Rafa ZI, Haque SN, et al. The Impact of Tezepelumab in Uncontrolled Severe Asthma: A Systematic Review of Randomized Controlled Trials. Cureus 2022;14(12):e32156.

Promising New Diagnostic and Treatment Modalities for Allergic Rhinitis
What's Coming Next?

Thomas F. Barrett, MD, Lauren T. Roland, MD, MSCI*

KEYWORDS

- Diagnosis • Testing • Allergic rhinitis • Research gaps

KEY POINTS

- Nasal allergen-specific IgE testing may help distinguish patients with local allergic rhinitis from patients with non-allergic rhinitis.
- Surgical techniques–including septoplasty, inferior turbinate reduction, nasal swell body reduction, and posterior nasal nerve ablation–often improve symptoms associated with allergic rhinitis in patients who are refractory to medical therapy.
- Epicutaneous and intralymphatic immunotherapy have the potential to decrease the logistical burdens of subcutaneous immunotherapy, but evidence is lacking to support their widespread adoption currently.

INTRODUCTION

Allergic rhinitis (AR) is among the most commonly encountered chronic conditions in high-income countries and it affects up to 50% of the population in some nations.[1] For the vast majority of patients, history and physical examination are sufficient to suggest the diagnosis of AR and begin empiric therapy with topical nasal steroids and possibly oral antihistamines.[2] For patients who do not respond to therapy, whose diagnosis remains uncertain, or who are seeking targeted therapy, either skin testing or *in vitro* serum specific IgE (sIgE) testing can be performed. The recent International Consensus Statement on Allergy and Rhinology: Allergic Rhinitis 2023 (ICAR:AR 2023) article provides a comprehensive overview of the recommendations for diagnosis and treatment for AR, based on the currently available literature.[3] Through a subject-specific systematic review, grading of the literature by level of evidence,

Division of Rhinology & Anterior Skull Base Surgery, Department of Otolaryngology–Head and Neck Surgery, Washington University School of Medicine, 660 South Euclid Avenue, St Louis, MO 63110, USA
* Correspondence author.
E-mail address: rolandl@wustl.edu

Otolaryngol Clin N Am 57 (2024) 243–251
https://doi.org/10.1016/j.otc.2023.08.008
0030-6665/24/© 2023 Elsevier Inc. All rights reserved.

and blinded iterative review process of all content, the document contains recommendations for both diagnosis and treatment. However, there are several new potential modalities on the way, which will require further evaluation, testing, and critical review prior to recommendation for widespread clinical use. Some of these are currently utilized for research purposes but may be clinically useful in the future. Several of these promising tools are described below.

DISCUSSION
Improved Diagnostics

Nitric oxide
Fractional exhaled nitric oxide (FeNO) is the measured NO in oral breath. This level can have a wide range in healthy patients. This test is most useful in asthmatics, and some work has suggested it may play a role in AR diagnosis.[3] Nasal nitric oxide (nNO) is measured by chemiluminescence and may be elevated in AR.[3] At this point, ICAR:AR recommends against routine use of these tests for AR diagnosis due to high cost, lack of sufficient evidence, and lack of an agreed upon cut-off value for diagnostic purposes.[3]

Nasal allergen-specific IgE
IgE-expressing B cells are 1,000 times more abundant in nasal B cell populations compared to peripheral blood populations, and allergens can stimulate local class switch recombination to IgE in the nasal mucosa.[4] Local sampling of nasal secretions through lavage, or sampling of mucosal tissue through biopsy or cytology brush, offers a potential means to directly sample sIgE that is locally expressed and secreted.[5] At the moment, the clinical utility of nasal allergen sIgE testing is most useful for those patients whose clinical history is strongly suggestive of AR but whose objective testing for systemic atopy (ie, skin testing and serum sIgE *in vitro* testing) has been negative.[6,7] Up to 1 in 4 patients with non-allergic rhinitis may actually have local AR (LAR). Patients with negative testing by conventional methods would typically not be offered allergy immunotherapy (AIT) treatment; however, limited and early studies have suggested that AIT improves symptoms in this population of patients.[8] A consensus on AIT in the LAR but otherwise negative-testing population is warranted. Additionally, standardization of nasal sIgE abnormal cut-off levels for consideration of diagnosis of AR has not been finalized.[3] This is an area of future potential research.

Basophil activation testing
Basophil activation testing (BAT) is a flow cytometry–based assay that measures the surface expression of activation markers (eg, CD63 and CD203c) on basophils after exposure to specific allergen extracts. As such, it is a more precise test than measuring serum sIgE.[9] While BAT is most commonly used in the setting of food, medication, and insect venom allergies, it has excellent sensitivity to house dust mite and grass pollen allergy in both adults and children.[9–11] However, its utility in monitoring of clinical responses to allergy immunotherapy (AIT) has been inconsistent across studies.[12,13] While BAT may have a role in distinguishing LAR from non-allergic rhinitis, further evidence is needed to support its broader clinical implementation.[3]

Rhinometry, acoustic rhinometry, and peak nasal inspiratory flow
While the diagnosis of AR can be made by clinical history with or without skin prick test (SPT) or sIgE levels in most cases, quantitative measures that correlate to patient symptoms are not yet widely adopted. Peak nasal inspiratory/expiratory flow (PNIF/PNEF) is a low-cost and easy-to-quantify measure. It is performed by placing an inspiratory flow meter connected to a pediatric cushioned face mask over the patient's nose. A minimal clinically important difference of 20 L/min or 20% after decongestion

has been described, and patients who do not achieve this response with medical therapy should be evaluated for structural causes of nasal obstruction.[14] Additional studies are needed to standardize these measures as patient confounders may potentially affect results. Confounders may include pulmonary status, nasal valve collapse, smoking status, stature, and patient effort. PNIF/PNEF should be considered an option as objective measures for response to therapy for AR in addition to standardized subjective instruments.[15]

Rhinomanometry refers to the measure of nasal airflow resistance (eg, the relationships between nasal airway pressure and flow). While classically rhinomanometry assessed flow at 150 Pa, 4-phase rhinomanometry (4PR) has been developed to assess nasal airflow in 4 distinct points in the nasal respiratory cycle: accelerating inspiratory phase, decelerating inspiratory phase, accelerating expiratory phase, and decelerating expiratory phase.[16] Rhinomanometry measures each side individually, and therefore it is not applicable in patients with nasal septal perforation or with complete unilateral obstruction. Limitations of the technique include its cost and the need for trained technicians to administer the testing.[17]

Acoustic rhinometry measures cross-sectional area and volume through acoustic reflections captured at various distances from the nasal inlet.[18] Importantly, acoustic rhinometry can suggest the site of obstruction. However, acoustic rhinometry is a static measurement and does not capture the dynamics of nasal airflow.

While more commonly used in the research setting at this point, these measures may prove to be useful as clinical diagnostic and treatment monitoring tools in the future.

Next-Line Therapeutics

For the majority of patients, the mainstays of medical management of AR consist of exposure modification (eg, allergen avoidance, environmental controls), topical nasal medications (eg, nasal saline, intranasal corticosteroids, intranasal antihistamines), and oral antihistamines. For patients with specific allergies whose symptoms do not respond to these conservative measures, AIT remains a highly effective option, provided the patient is able to make the time and financial commitment. This section will discuss advances in the surgical management in AR, novel implementations of AIT, and adjuncts to AIT.

Surgical procedures for allergic rhinitis

When patients fail conservative medical management, surgery may provide benefit, either through correction of anatomic causes of nasal airway obstruction, or by directly altering the physiologic cause of symptoms. Potential structural targets of surgery are the nasal septum, the inferior turbinate, and the nasal swell body (NSB). Physiologic targets include the vidian nerve and one of its terminal branches, the posterior nasal nerve.

AR patients with significant obstructive nasal symptoms may benefit from septoplasty, with or without inferior turbinate reduction (ITR).[19] Septoplasty is most appropriate for patients who have failed conservative medical management and have a septal deviation that is present on either anterior rhinoscopy or nasal endoscopy. Septoplasty may be performed through a traditional transnasal approach, endoscopically, or as part of an open septorhinoplasty.[20,21] It should be noted that studies to support septoplasty in the AR population have included mixed populations of patients, and that studies primarily evaluating the benefit of septoplasty for AR are lacking.[22] Furthermore, the evidence consists largely of case series and subjective quality of life (QOL) measures are most commonly reported.

ITR, however, is better studied in the AR population. Existing studies report improvement in rhinitis-related symptoms, including nasal breathing, congestion, sneezing, and itching.[23,24] It is postulated that, in addition to reducing nasal obstruction and minimizing the impact of reactive mucosal swelling, ITR also decreases the overall surface area of mucosa that may potentially react with allergens. Multiple techniques exist, including a simple outfracture,[25] submucosal resection,[26] and energy-related techniques (eg, radiofrequency reduction),[27] although no technique has demonstrated clear benefit relative to others.

The NSB, sometimes referred to as the nasal septal turbinate, is a fusiform region of the anterior nasal septum composed of cartilage, bone, and thickened mucosa and contains vasoactive tissue. Volumetric reduction of the NSB with various techniques (including radiofrequency ablation, laser, and coblation) has been proposed as an additional intervention to improve nasal airflow.[28,29] Several devices designed for use in either the clinic or the operating room have come to market (eg, Vivaer from Aerin Medical), though evidence to support their use specifically in AR is lacking.

To some extent, rhinorrhea associated with AR is mediated by parasympathetic innervation via the vidian nerve and its distal branches. Vidian neurectomy is an effective approach to improve sneezing, nasal discharge, nasal obstruction, itching, and several QOL measures, though not without significant risk for ipsilateral lifelong dry eye.[30,31] Targeting more distal parasympathetic branches of the vidian has shown great potential to avoid this troublesome side effect.[32] In particular, targeting the posterior nasal nerve with either radio frequency (RF) energy–based ablation (Rhinaer, Aerin Medical) or cryoablation (Clarifix, Stryker) has shown benefit in a number of conditions associated with rhinorrhea.[33] While no study has specifically compared these techniques in patients with AR, subgroup analyses within the existing studies suggest that AR patients' rhinorrhea improves. A randomized sham-controlled clinical trial suggested that RF ablation is effective.[34] Overall, these procedures appear to be well-tolerated and bear minimal complication risk. Most existing studies, however, have been industry-sponsored with little long-term follow-up. Future work in this area should be focused on evaluating the safety and cost-effectiveness of these surgical interventions specifically for AR.[3]

Epicutaneous immunotherapy

Epicutaneous immunotherapy is a non-invasive form of AIT that consists of application of allergens to the skin.[3] This method may be preferred in that it does not require injections, and AIT is delivered through skin patches.[3] Several techniques for delivery of antigen have been trialed including tape stripping, abrasion of the skin, and sweat accumulation through patch application.[3,35,36] Powder-based AIT has also been attempted into the epidermis using microneedle arrays and laser-mediated microporation.[37] Unfortunately, there is very limited evidence on this AIT delivery mechanism for AR due to inhalant allergy. Evidence to date for AR is limited to multiple single-center double-blind randomized control trials comparing grass patches to placebo patches.[38] There have not been any head-to-head comparisons with the widely used delivery mechanisms, subcutaneous immunotherapy (SCIT) or sublingual immunotherapy (SLIT).

The limited existing evidence has shown mixed benefits, and due to lack of available data, extensive statistical analysis has not been done. Unfortunately, both local and systemic reactions are common with epicutaneous immunotherapy. At this point, the ICAR:AR document recommends against this option;[3] however, in theory, this is a promising modality to improve convenience of AIT. If determined to be a safe option, epicutaneous delivery may prove to be convenient for both children and adults, avoiding weekly injections and clinic visits associated with SCIT, and potentially avoiding the oral and gastrointestinal side effects of SLIT.

Intralymphatic immunotherapy (ILIT)

Another potential future method of AIT is ILIT. This method requires ultrasound-guided injection of low-dose allergens directly into lymph nodes. Inguinal and cervical lymph nodes have been utilized.[3,39] ILIT, while an invasive treatment, has a very short treatment duration. The tested protocols have generally used approximately 3 injections over a period of only 2 months.[40] If able to reach clinical improvement in a short time, this delivery mechanism may be preferred by select patients.

There has been limited work done regarding ILIT. While local side effects were higher in ILIT compared to placebo, the overall rate of systemic and local side effects are thought to be lower in ILIT administration compared to SCIT.[41] There have not been any studies directly comparing ILIT to SLIT.[3] Unfortunately, while short-term improvement has been documented, long-term efficacy has not been well established from limited ILIT studies.[40,42] Prior to incorporation into practice, long-term efficacy will need to be determined.

Oral, nasal, and inhaled routes of allergy immunotherapy administration

Multiple other administration techniques for AIT are under investigation and may prove to be useful as treatment options in the future. These methods are early in their development and require further study for tolerance, efficacy, and cost-effectiveness. Some options include oral, nasal, and inhaled administration, allowing allergens to be absorbed into the oral, GI, nasal, or bronchial mucosa.[3] Oral administration of AIT requires high doses at this point and is associated with GI side effects.[3,43] Therefore, while

Table 1
Limitations to be addressed prior to widespread use of potential new diagnostic and treatment modalities

Potential Diagnostic Tool or Treatment for AR	Current Limitations to be Addressed
Nitric oxide	• High cost • Lack of established cut-off values for diagnosis
Nasal allergen-specific IgE	• Standardization of cut-off value for diagnosis
Basophil activation test	• Evaluation of sensitivity of additional allergens for clinical use
Peak nasal flow	• Standardization of measurement
Rhinometry	• Cost • Training • Need for evaluation of dynamic flow
Surgical procedures	• Cost-effectiveness analyses for AR specifically
Epicutaneous immunotherapy	• Further safety evaluation • Comparison to SLIT and SCIT for safety and efficacy
Intralymphatic immunotherapy	• Evaluation of long-term efficacy • Comparison to SLIT and SCIT for safety and efficacy
Oral, nasal, and inhaled Immunotherapy	• Further work for improved safety and tolerance
Combination (biologics and SCIT)	• Cost-effectiveness analyses to determine clear indications

effective for food allergies, oral AIT has not yet been adopted for AR treatment and requires future work.[44] Oral mucosal delivery mechanisms (such as toothpaste) are another potential administration option. There has been limited work on this mechanism, and efficacy has not been definitively confirmed.[45] Local nasal AIT has been studied for select antigens,however, this treatment has not been well tolerated.[46] Further work is needed to determine the role of inhaled/bronchial delivery of AIT for AR.[3]

Combination biologic + subcutaneous immunotherapy

While 3 biologics have been approved for use in patients with chronic rhinosinusitis with nasal polyps, biologics have not been approved for use in AR. However, several studies have evaluated omalizumab (anti-IgE) as either a standalone or adjunct therapy with AIT for treatment of AR.[47] At this point, anti-IgE therapy has been suggested to improve tolerance for cluster or rush SCIT protocols. A phase 2a double-blind randomized controlled trial comparing SCIT, dupilumab, SCIT and dupilumab, and placebo found that dupilumab may improve tolerance of SCIT, but did not improve symptom scores during post-treatment allergen challenge.[3,48] Additionally, biologics may be helpful in select patients with continued AR symptoms despite AIT.[3] Further work is necessary to determine efficacy and indications of combination biologic therapy as well as cost-effectiveness for this medication class in AR.

SUMMARY

Novel diagnostic tests–including nasal allergen-specific IgE and basophil activation testing–may help differentiate patients with LAR. Surgical approaches including septoplasty, ITR, NSB reduction, and posterior nasal nerve ablation may improve symptoms in patients whose symptoms are refractory to medical therapy, though high-quality evidence is lacking in the AR population. Intralymphatic and epicutaneous immunotherapy have potential to improve adherence to AIT, though head-to-head comparisons with current standard of care treatments are lacking and studies reporting long-term outcomes are needed. Immunomodulatory agents in combination with SCIT may improve tolerance of SCIT but reports to date do not demonstrate a clear benefit in symptom alleviation. Future research should focus on these potential and promising diagnostic and testing options to advance the field of AR (**Table 1**).

DISCLOSURE

The authors have no relevant disclosures.

REFERENCES

1. Bousquet J, Anto JM, Bachert C, et al. Allergic rhinitis. Nat Rev Dis Primers 2020; 6(1):95.
2. Seidman MD, Gurgel RK, Lin SY, et al. Clinical Practice Guideline: Allergic Rhinitis. Otolaryngol Head Neck Surg 2015;152(S1). https://doi.org/10.1177/0194599814561600.
3. Wise SK, Damask C, Roland LT, et al. International consensus statement on allergy and rhinology: Allergic rhinitis – 2023. Int Forum Allergy Rhinol 2023; 13(4):293–859.
4. Takhar P, Smurthwaite L, Coker HA, et al. Allergen Drives Class Switching to IgE in the Nasal Mucosa in Allergic Rhinitis. J Immunol 2005;174(8):5024–32.
5. Hamizan A, Alvarado R, Rimmer J, et al. Nasal mucosal brushing as a diagnostic method for allergic rhinitis. Allergy Asthma Proc 2019;40(3):167–72.

6. Rondón C, Romero JJ, López S, et al. Local IgE production and positive nasal provocation test in patients with persistent nonallergic rhinitis. J Allergy Clin Immunol 2007;119(4):899–905.

7. Rondón C, Doña I, López S, et al. Seasonal idiopathic rhinitis with local inflammatory response and specific IgE in absence of systemic response. Allergy 2008;63(10):1352–8.

8. Eguiluz-Gracia I, Ariza A, Testera-Montes A, et al. Allergen Immunotherapy for Local Respiratory Allergy. Curr Allergy Asthma Rep 2020;20(7):23.

9. Santos AF, Alpan O, Hoffmann H. Basophil activation test: Mechanisms and considerations for use in clinical trials and clinical practice. Allergy 2021;76(8):2420–32.

10. Ogulur I, Kiykim A, Baris S, et al. Basophil activation test for inhalant allergens in pediatric patients with allergic rhinitis. Int J Pediatr Otorhinolaryngol 2017;97:197–201.

11. Özdemir SK, Güloğlu D, Sin BA, et al. Reliability of basophil activation test using CD203c expression in diagnosis of pollen allergy. Am J Rhinol Allergy 2011;25(6):e225–31.

12. Feng M, Zeng X, Su Q, et al. Allergen Immunotherapy-Induced Immunoglobulin G4 Reduces Basophil Activation in House Dust Mite-Allergic Asthma Patients. Front Cell Dev Biol 2020;8:30.

13. Aasbjerg K, Backer V, Lund G, et al. Immunological comparison of allergen immunotherapy tablet treatment and subcutaneous immunotherapy against grass allergy. Clin Exp Allergy 2014;44(3):417–28.

14. Timperley D, Srubisky A, Stow N, et al. Minimal clinically important differences in nasal peak inspiratory flow. Rhinology 2011;49(1):37–40.

15. Kirtsreesakul V, Leelapong J, Ruttanaphol S. Nasal peak inspiratory and expiratory flow measurements for assessing nasal obstruction in allergic rhinitis. Am J Rhinol Allergy 2014;28(2):126–30.

16. Vogt K, Wernecke KD, Behrbohm H, et al. Four-phase rhinomanometry: a multicentric retrospective analysis of 36,563 clinical measurements. Eur Arch Oto-Rhino-Laryngol 2016;273(5):1185–98.

17. André RF, Vuyk HD, Ahmed A, et al. Correlation between subjective and objective evaluation of the nasal airway. A systematic review of the highest level of evidence. Clin Otolaryngol 2009;34(6):518–25.

18. Uzzaman A, Metcalfe DD, Komarow HD. Acoustic rhinometry in the practice of allergy. Ann Allergy Asthma Immunol 2006;97(6):745–51, quiz 751-752, 799.

19. Karatzanis AD, Fragiadakis G, Moshandrea J, et al. Septoplasty outcome in patients with and without allergic rhinitis. Rhinology 2009;47(4):444–9.

20. Sokoya M, Gonzalez JR, Winkler AA. Effect of allergic rhinitis on nasal obstruction outcomes after functional open septorhinoplasty. Am J Otolaryngol 2018;39(3):303–6.

21. Gerecci D, Casanueva FJ, Mace JC, et al. Nasal obstruction symptom evaluation (NOSE) score outcomes after septorhinoplasty. Laryngoscope 2019;129(4):841–6.

22. Gillman GS, Staltari GV, Chang YF, et al. A Prospective Study of Outcomes of Septoplasty with Turbinate Reductions in Patients with Allergic Rhinitis. Otolaryngol Head Neck Surg 2019;160(6):1118–23.

23. Huang TW, Cheng PW. Changes in nasal resistance and quality of life after endoscopic microdebrider-assisted inferior turbinoplasty in patients with perennial allergic rhinitis. Arch Otolaryngol Head Neck Surg 2006;132(9):990–3.

24. Liu CM, Tan CD, Lee FP, et al. Microdebrider-assisted versus radiofrequency-assisted inferior turbinoplasty. Laryngoscope 2009;119(2):414–8.
25. Sinno S, Mehta K, Lee ZH, et al. Inferior Turbinate Hypertrophy in Rhinoplasty: Systematic Review of Surgical Techniques. Plast Reconstr Surg 2016;138(3):419e–29e.
26. Ghosh SK, Dutta M, Haldar D. Role of Bilateral Inferior Turbinoplasty as an Adjunct to Septoplasty in Improving Nasal Obstruction and Subjective Performance in Patients With Deviated Nasal Septum Associated With Allergic Rhinitis: An Interventional, Prospective Study. Ear Nose Throat J 2023;102(7):445–52.
27. Kang T, Sung CM, Yang HC. Radiofrequency ablation of turbinates after septoplasty has no effect on allergic rhinitis symptoms other than nasal obstruction. Int Forum Allergy Rhinol 2019;9(11):1257–62.
28. Krespi YP, Wilson KA, Kizhner V. Nasal nerve ablation, nasal swell body and inferior turbinate reduction for nasal obstruction and congestion relief. J Laryngol Otol 2023;137(3):270–2.
29. Kim SJ, Kim HT, Park YH, et al. Coblation nasal septal swell body reduction for treatment of nasal obstruction: a preliminary report. Eur Arch Oto-Rhino-Laryngol 2016;273(9):2575–8.
30. Maimaitiaili G, Kahaer K, Tang L, et al. The Effect of Vidian Neurectomy on Pulmonary Function in Patients with Allergic Rhinitis and Chronic Rhinosinusitis with Nasal Polyps. Am J Med Sci 2020;360(2):137–45.
31. Shen L, Wang J, Kang X, et al. Clinical Efficacy and Possible Mechanism of Endoscopic Vidian Neurectomy for House Dust Mite-Sensitive Allergic Rhinitis. ORL J Otorhinolaryngol Relat Spec 2021;83(2):75–84.
32. Wang L, Chen M, Xu M. Effect of posterior nasal neurectomy on the suppression of allergic rhinitis. Am J Otolaryngol 2020;41(3):102410.
33. Lee ML, Chakravarty PD, Ellul D. Posterior nasal neurectomy for intractable rhinitis: A systematic review of the literature. Clin Otolaryngol 2023;48(2):95–107.
34. Stolovitzky JP, Ow RA, Silvers SL, et al. Effect of Radiofrequency Neurolysis on the Symptoms of Chronic Rhinitis: A Randomized Controlled Trial. OTO Open 2021;5(3). 2473974X211041124.
35. Gunawardana NC, Durham SR. New approaches to allergen immunotherapy. Ann Allergy Asthma Immunol 2018;121(3):293–305.
36. Senti G, Kündig TM. Novel Delivery Routes for Allergy Immunotherapy: Intralymphatic, Epicutaneous, and Intradermal. Immunol Allergy Clin North Am 2016;36(1):25–37.
37. Wang Y, Kong Y, Wu MX. Innovative Systems to Deliver Allergen Powder for Epicutaneous Immunotherapy. Front Immunol 2021;12:647954.
38. Senti G, von Moos S, Tay F, et al. Determinants of efficacy and safety in epicutaneous allergen immunotherapy: summary of three clinical trials. Allergy 2015;70(6):707–10.
39. Senti G, Freiburghaus AU, Larenas-Linnemann D, et al. Intralymphatic Immunotherapy: Update and Unmet Needs. Int Arch Allergy Immunol 2019;178(2):141–9.
40. Hoang MP, Seresirikachorn K, Chitsuthipakorn W, et al. Intralymphatic immunotherapy for allergic rhinoconjunctivitis: a systematic review and meta-analysis. Rhinology 2021;59(3):236–44.
41. Senti G, Prinz Vavricka BM, Erdmann I, et al. Intralymphatic allergen administration renders specific immunotherapy faster and safer: a randomized controlled trial. Proc Natl Acad Sci U S A 2008;105(46):17908–12.

42. Aini NR, Mohd Noor N, Md Daud MK, et al. Efficacy and safety of intralymphatic immunotherapy in allergic rhinitis: A systematic review and meta-analysis. Clin Transl Allergy 2021;11(6):e12055.
43. Cox L, Nelson H, Lockey R, et al. Allergen immunotherapy: a practice parameter third update. J Allergy Clin Immunol 2011;127(1 Suppl):S1–55.
44. PALISADE Group of Clinical Investigators, Vickery BP, Vereda A, et al. AR101 Oral Immunotherapy for Peanut Allergy. N Engl J Med 2018;379(21):1991–2001.
45. Reisacher WR, Suurna MV, Rochlin K, et al. Oral mucosal immunotherapy for allergic rhinitis: A pilot study. Allergy Rhinol (Providence) 2016;7(1):21–8.
46. Pajno GB, Vita D, Caminiti L, et al. Children's compliance with allergen immuno-therapy according to administration routes. J Allergy Clin Immunol 2005;116(6):1380–1.
47. Tsabouri S, Ntritsos G, Koskeridis F, et al. Omalizumab for the treatment of allergic rhinitis: a systematic review and meta-analysis. Rhinology 2021;59(6):501–10.
48. Corren J, Saini SS, Gagnon R, et al. Short-Term Subcutaneous Allergy Immuno-therapy and Dupilumab are Well Tolerated in Allergic Rhinitis: A Randomized Trial. J Asthma Allergy 2021;14:1045–63.

Allergy and Asthma Prevalence and Management Across Nasal Polyp Subtypes

Kody G. Bolk, MD*, Thomas S. Edwards, MD,
Sarah K. Wise, MD, MSCR, John M. DelGaudio, MD

KEYWORDS

- Allergy • Asthma • Chronic sinusitis • Nasal polyps • Allergic fungal rhinosinusitis
- Central compartment atopic disease • Aspirin-exacerbated respiratory disease

KEY POINTS

- Numerous endotypes make up the phenotype of nasal polyps, and the prevalence of asthma and allergy varies widely across endotypes.
- There is limited, and often conflicting, evidence regarding the role that allergy management has on different nasal polyp subtypes.
- Treatment that accounts for both upper and lower airway effects of disease leads to improved overall outcomes.

INTRODUCTION

Chronic rhinosinusitis (CRS) affects approximately 4.5% to 12% of the population of the United States and European countries.[1–3] It is usually divided into categories of CRS with nasal polyps (CRSwNP) and CRS without nasal polyps. CRSwNP affects about 2.1% to 4.3% of people.[4] Efforts to further classify CRS based on inflammatory profile, or endotype, are ongoing. Generally, T-helper (Th) type 1 inflammation is mediated by interleukin (IL)-12 and interferon gamma, creating neutrophil driven inflammation. Th2 inflammation is mediated by IL-4, IL-5, and IL-13, and the inflammation is influenced by immunoglobulin (Ig) E. Th17/22 is mediated by IL-17 and IL-22, which promote neutrophil and macrophage response.[5–9]

The association of CRS with other common upper and lower respiratory tract inflammatory disorders, allergic rhinitis (AR), and asthma has long been questioned. While the inflammatory signatures of certain endotypes of CRS do seem to provide a plausible biologic basis for an association, numerous clinical studies have revealed

Department of Otolaryngology–Head and Neck Surgery, Emory University Hospital Midtown, 550 Peachtree Street NE, MOT Suite 1135, Atlanta, GA 30308, USA
* Corresponding author.
E-mail address: kodybolk@gmail.com

Otolaryngol Clin N Am 57 (2024) 253–263
https://doi.org/10.1016/j.otc.2023.09.001
0030-6665/24/© 2023 Elsevier Inc. All rights reserved.

oto.theclinics.com

contradictory findings.[10] In this section, the authors discuss the various nasal polyp subtypes and their interaction with asthma and AR.

Chronic Rhinosinusitis, Allergy, and Asthma

CRS is an inflammatory condition affecting the nasal cavity and paranasal sinuses. It is characterized by symptoms of nasal discharge, nasal obstruction, hyposmia, and facial pain/pressure lasting for more than 12 weeks. There must also be objective evidence of inflammation with endoscopic findings of edema and/or mucopurulence or computed tomography (CT) suggestive of chronic inflammation.[7,11]

Individuals affected by inhalant allergy produce IgE antibodies against environmental allergens. The development of atopy to these triggers is a complex mechanism composed of many factors including indoor and outdoor exposures, chemical exposures, host genetic factors and age, and timing of exposure that interplay together.[12] Individuals with allergy have a hypersensitivity reaction on exposure to an antigen that usually would not produce symptoms in nonallergic individuals. In AR, this results in the classic symptoms of allergy: nasal drainage, nasal obstruction, nasal itching, and/or sneezing.[7,13]

Asthma is an inflammatory condition of the bronchi and bronchioles of the lungs leading to episodic obstruction and symptoms of dyspnea, cough, and wheezing.[14] There have been endotypes and phenotypes described for asthma. The endotypes are based on the presence or absence of Th2 cytokines and are described as type 2 high and type 2 low asthma. Phenotypes include atopic, late onset, and aspirin-exacerbated respiratory disease (AERD), which are primarily mediated by type 2 inflammation. Other phenotypic subtypes include nonatopic, smoking-related, obesity-related, and very late-onset or elderly, which are non-type 2–mediated subtypes of asthma. Atopic asthma is driven by allergic sensitization and biomarkers include elevated IgE.[15,16]

Allergic sensitization is a significant risk factor for asthma.[17] There is strong evidence showing that control of AR is beneficial in patients with allergic asthma, reducing short-term symptoms and medication scores.[18] In a meta-analysis by Dhami and colleagues in 2017, patients treated with subcutaneous immunotherapy had improvement in asthma-specific quality of life and reduction in allergen-specific airway hyperreactivity. However, there was no significant change in asthma control with allergen immunotherapy. Additionally, there were asthma exacerbations, but no fatalities, noted with immunotherapy.[17]

Type 2 Inflammation

Allergy and some forms of asthma and CRS share a common link in pathogenesis via type 2 inflammation. This includes elevated levels of inflammatory mediators like IL-4, IL-5, and IL-13.[19,20] Antigen presenting cells activate Th2 cells to produce IL-4, IL-13, and IL-5. These mediators recruit mast cells, eosinophils, basophils, and goblet cells, M2 macrophages, and B cells throughout the upper and lower airway.[1,7] This leads to increased IgE production and eosinophilia as well as heightened responsiveness to allergens. Histamine release leads to flushing, edema, nasal congestion, and bronchospasm. Prostaglandin D2 causes smooth muscle contraction with bronchoconstriction, and cysteinyl leukotriene causes nasal congestion, rhinorrhea, and loss of smell.[1]

ALLERGY AND ASTHMA ACROSS CHRONIC RHINOSINUSITIS WITH NASAL POLYPS SUBTYPES

Twenty-seven percent to 75% of all adults and children with asthma have concurrent rhinosinusitis.[1,21–24] About 25% to 58% of individuals with CRS have aeroallergen sensitization.[25] This increases to 76% for patients with CRSwNP.[26] Patients with certain types of CRS, asthma, and/or allergy show benefit when treated for the comorbid condition(s).[27]

Asthma and allergy have been shown to be interconnected as well. Asthma is present in about 15% to 30% of patients with AR, and AR is present in a large majority of patients with asthma, up to 90% by some estimates.[28]

Prior research has shown that inflammation in the nasal mucosa and lower airways is directly related. In patients with severe asthma, the extent of sinonasal disease present on imaging correlates with airway inflammation measured by bronchial or serum eosinophil levels.[1] Studies have shown improvement in asthma scores following endoscopic sinus surgery (ESS) in patients with CRSwNP. This includes improved asthma control scores and decreased numbers of asthma attacks and hospitalizations.[26,29] There are also improvements in objective asthma measures as well as reductions in hospitalizations and bronchodilator and oral steroid use.[29] A 2020 study by Hamada and colleagues demonstrated that these impacts were durable. Patients with asthma and CRSwNP had improvement in asthma control questionnaires and improved spirometry 1 year after ESS. There was suppression of both airway and systemic type 2 inflammation leading to improvement.[24]

Also, it has been shown that eosinophilia in nasal tissue as well as fractional exhaled nitric oxide (FeNO) measurements may help to determine which patients with CRS are likely to develop asthma, with higher tissue eosinophilia and elevated FeNO increasing likelihood.[30] Interestingly, it does not appear that all asthma patients with CRSwNP behave similarly. Birs and colleagues noted that different phenotypes of asthma, such as the evolution of onset, exist in the CRSwNP population.[31] In patient with CRSwNP, asthma onset may occur later, suggesting a possible unique mechanism for this asthma subtype.[32] Further exploration of these asthma subtypes may help to optimize treatment for these patients.[31,32]

Table 1 shows the various subtypes of CRSwNP and the associated characteristics of the disease, prevalence of allergy and asthma, as well as the management strategies.

Aspirin-exacerbated Respiratory Disease

AERD is a subtype of CRSwNP. This diagnosis is typically made when patients have asthma, nasal polyposis, and respiratory sensitivity to aspirin or nonsteroidal anti-inflammatory drugs.[4,6] AERD affects 0.3% to 0.9% of the population, 10% to 20% of asthmatics, and 30% to 40% of asthmatics with nasal polyps.[33] These patients have abnormal arachidonic acid metabolism. When cyclo-oxygenase (COX)-1 inhibitors are introduced, cysteinyl leukotrienes are produced and there is a reduction in prostaglandin E2 production leading to increased production of leukotriene E4. This leads to recruitment of eosinophils and results in type 2 inflammatory respiratory symptoms.[4,34–36] This is a non-IgE mediated hypersensitivity to the COX-1 inhibitors.[37] As asthma is part of the diagnostic criteria for AERD, 100% of AERD patients have asthma. The gold standard for AERD diagnosis is aspirin challenge. AERD patients will usually have pansinus opacification on CT imaging as well.[33]

Many AERD patients exhibit atopy.[13,38] In a study by DelGaudio and colleagues, AR prevalence in AERD patients was 89.9%.[38] In this study, 72 AERD patients were examined, and 59 patients had central compartment involvement of their disease. Of the AERD patients with central compartment disease, 93.8% showed sensitivity to at least 1 allergen on testing. Interestingly, only 42.8% of AERD patients without central compartment involvement were noted to have positive allergy testing.[38] An additional study by Bochenek and colleagues noted in their AERD cohort that 52%

Table 1
Characteristics and management of nasal polyp subtypes

	AERD	AFRS	CCAD
Disease characteristics	Asthma, nasal polyposis, respiratory sensitivity to ASA or NSAIDs	Nasal polyposis, fungal elements on stain, characteristic radiographic findings, eosinophilic mucin without fungal invasion, type 1 hypersensitivity to fungi	Nasal obstruction, polypoid changes of central nasal cavity including posterior/superior nasal septum and middle/superior turbinates, low prevalence of asthma
Allergy prevalence	36%–89.9%	100%	74%–100%
Asthma prevalence	100%	11.4%–30.8%	17%
Primary management strategies for nasal polyposis	ESS, intranasal steroids, saline irrigations, leukotriene-modifying medications, biologic therapies, ASA desensitization	ESS, intranasal steroids, saline irrigations, allergen immunotherapy (consideration), biologic therapies (actively under investigation)	ESS of involved central disease, intranasal steroids, saline irrigations, allergen immunotherapy (consideration)

Abbreviations: AERD, aspirin-exacerbated respiratory disease; AFRS, allergic fungal rhinosinusitis; ASA, acetylsalicylic acid; CCAD, central compartment atopic disease; ESS, endoscopic sinus surgery; NSAIDs, nonsteroidal anti-inflammatory drugs.

has positive skin prick testing.[39] Other studies have noted prevalence between 36% and 66%.[40–42]

Management options for AERD include aspirin desensitization with continued daily aspirin therapy or complete avoidance of COX-1 inhibitors. The benefits of high-dose daily aspirin, usually 650 mg twice daily, include improvement in nasal polyp scores, reduced need for sinus surgery, improved sense of smell, decreased use of steroids, and reduction in sinus infections.[33,43,44] However, a subset of patients, approximately 20%, do not have symptom control on aspirin therapy. Others are unable to continue therapy due to other medical contraindications or side effects.[44]

ESS is typically indicated for AERD patients, and their course is often recalcitrant, requiring multiple revision surgeries.[37] Other therapies include intranasal steroids and saline irrigations, and one may consider leukotriene-modifying drugs as well. Leukotriene-modifying drugs include 5-lipoxygenase inhibitors as well as leukotriene receptor antagonists. These have been utilized to help control lower airway symptoms and have been found to improve lung function, reduce bronchodilator use, reduce asthma exacerbations, and improve quality of life.[37,44]

Additional treatment considerations include biologic therapies. Omalizumab is a humanized recombinant monoclonal antibody therapy against IgE. AERD is not an IgE-mediated disease, but patients with aspirin sensitivity that have been treated with omalizumab for nasal polyps and asthma have seen improvements.[44] Dupilumab and mepolizumab are other monoclonal antibody therapies used to treat nasal polyps, but there have not been specific clinical trials for AERD. In the trials for efficacy of biologics for CRSwNP patients, between 17% and 39% of the patients in those cohorts had AERD on further analysis. These patients were noted to see improvements when treated with biologics in areas like nasal polyp score.[45] In patients with AERD treated with dupilumab, there have been reports of efficacy in treating nasal symptoms, nasal polyp burden, as well as lung function.[35,46,47] Additional study is needed to further evaluate efficacy in this population.[44]

In a study by Mullur and colleagues, 24 patients with AERD were treated with aspirin desensitization as well as biologic therapy. They noted these patients were moderate responders to aspirin desensitization, meaning they noted some benefits, but additional therapy in biologics was sought out due to remaining symptoms. These patients were noted to be older than others.[48] Another study proposes that biologics may be used as a step-up therapy if there is incomplete symptom control with aspirin desensitization. However, cost analysis may play a role in treatment options as well, with biologic therapy costing more than aspirin desensitization therapy.[49] Further research is necessary to determine if different phenotypes of AERD exist to help determine efficacy of aspirin desensitization or biologic therapy amongst patients.

Allergen immunotherapy has not been recommended for the standard treatment of AERD, and it has not been formally studied for this patient population. As it stands, these patients should be treated with immunotherapy if there is clear evidence of comorbid, seasonal, or perennial allergic symptoms in addition to CRS.[44]

Allergic Fungal Rhinosinusitis

Allergic fungal rhinosinusitis (AFRS) is another subtype of CRSwNP. The most commonly cited AFRS diagnostic criteria were published by Bent and Kuhn in 1994 with major criteria including nasal polyps, fungal elements present on staining, eosinophilic mucin without fungal invasion, type 1 hypersensitivity to fungi, and characteristic radiographic findings (unilaterally or asymmetric findings, bony remodeling, and heterogenous densities within the sinuses).[50] Minor criteria include bone erosion,

Charcot-Leyden crystals, unilateral disease, peripheral eosinophilia, positive fungal culture, and lack of immunodeficient state.[50,51] Patients usually present with symptoms of CRS including nasal obstruction, hyposmia/anosmia, facial pain/pressure, thick rhinorrhea, and possibly orbital proptosis or telecanthus.[7] Endoscopy may show diffuse nasal polyposis with thick yellow/brown mucin.[7] Interestingly, these patients present at a younger age and in geographic regions with warm temperatures and high humidity.[52,53]

Comorbid asthma and AR can exist in this cohort.[6] A study by Xu and colleagues noted 51.4% of patients diagnosed with AFRS had signs and symptoms of AR and 11.4% had signs and symptoms of asthma.[52] Asthma prevalence has been noted to be up to 30.8%.[6,54] Marcus and colleagues noted that in the AFRS cohort of patients, 100% had positive allergy testing and 19% had comorbid asthma.[6] AFRS is mediated by a type 2 immune response.[52] A study by Luong and colleagues noted that exposure to fungal antigens stimulated a predominantly Th2-type response in patients with AFRS.[55] This is similar to the mechanism seen in allergy and certain subtypes of asthma. In a study by Promsopa and colleagues using pulmonary function testing, asthma was present in 23.6% of AFRS patients. Asthma was significantly less prevalent in the AFRS group than in the CRSwNP not otherwise specified group which had a prevalence of 48.3%. This may be due to differences in pathogenesis between AFRS and other types of CRSwNP.[20] It is theorized that a defect in the innate immune system by fungal protease–activated toll-like receptor-4 causes sinonasal and airway responsiveness to fungi. However, this pathway, when knocked out in mice, causes attenuation of the airway hyperreactivity but the adaptive Th2 response remains unaffected. This may help to explain the lower incidence of asthma in patients with AFRS.[56]

ESS is typically undertaken to remove nasal polyps and mucin. The natural ostia are opened widely to allow for postoperative sinonasal irrigation with topical corticosteroids. There may be a role for allergen immunotherapy, but this has not been well supported.[7] Mabry and colleagues studied 11 patients with AFRS treated by surgery initially, with immunotherapy initiated for fungal and nonfungal antigens to which they were sensitive. In the first 3 years, they noted no patients had adverse reactions to the treatment. None of the patients required systemic steroids and only 3 required intranasal steroids. No additional surgeries were required in this follow-up timeframe.[57–59] Further, when immunotherapy was discontinued for 8 patients in this cohort, there was no recurrence of symptoms at up to 17 months in follow-up.[60] A study by Doellman and colleagues summarized some of the literature on usage of immunotherapy in AFRS patients. Patient treated with surgery and then immunotherapy had lower steroid usage and surgeries after 3 years; however, longer term immunotherapy did not have significant improvement compared to controls.[61]

Biologic therapies have been used to treat patients with asthma and concurrent AFRS as well. These trials were not specifically for AFRS, but, interestingly, when biologics like omalizumab or mepolizumab have been utilized in patients with AFRS, there have been improvements in asthma scores like forced expiratory volume in 1 second, symptom scores, and quality of life, and decreased oral corticosteroid use.[46]

Central Compartment Atopic Disease

Central compartment atopic disease (CCAD) is characterized by polypoid changes of central nasal cavity including areas of the posterior/superior nasal septum, middle turbinates, and/or superior turbinate. These patients may present with symptoms of nasal obstruction, hyposmia/anosmia, facial pain/pressure, clear rhinorrhea as well as nasal itching and sneezing.[7,54]

This disease process has a strong association with allergy.[38] Prior studies have shown allergy sensitization in 74% to 100% of patients.[5,6] It is thought that nasal airflow through the central aspect of the nasal cavity causes allergen deposition in this region, and subsequent inflammatory change and polyposis. Asthma prevalence in this population is comparatively low, about 17%.[6,54,62]

Workup of CCAD frequently includes skin and in vitro IgE testing. There also may be a role for testing intranasal local allergens as prior studies have indicated some patients with a clinical picture of CCAD may have local sensitivity that is not present systemically.[5] CT imaging in early CCAD shows only central nasal cavity soft tissue thickening with sparing of the sinuses. As the central compartment disease progresses, the sinuses become involved as a result of postobstructive disease due to lateralization of the middle turbinates or polypoid degeneration of the lateral surface of the middle turbinates. In severe CCAD, the sinuses may show significant mucosal thickening or even complete opacification, making radiologic differentiation from other CRSwNP subtypes difficult. Oblique orientation of the middle turbinates (due to central compartment polyps) is a finding in severe CCAD.[7,62]

Endoscopic surgery is utilized to sculpt the central compartment by removing polypoid changes in CCAD. The sinuses should be addressed surgically when they are involved, but uninvolved sinuses should be left unoperated in order to reduce exposure to inhaled antigens. Topical corticosteroid irrigations are typically used. Immunotherapy has been suggested as an adjunct treatment as well, but its role is currently not well studied.[4,7] Other medical therapies may include topical antihistamines and oral antihistamines, but further clinical investigation is necessary.[5] Studies on the impact of allergen immunotherapy as well as other medical therapies for AR on treatment outcomes in patients with CCAD are needed.

FUTURE DIRECTIONS

Several monoclonal antibody therapies that target Th2 inflammation are now available. Dupilumab is an anti-IL-4 alpha receptor monoclonal antibody which inhibits both IL-4 and IL-13. This has shown efficacy in treating CRSwNP as well as asthma.[1] In a study by Laidlaw and colleagues, patients with AERD treated with dupilumab had improved nasal polyp scores, sinonasal outcome test-22 (SNOT-22) scores, and asthma control questionnaire scores at 16 weeks.[47] Omalizumab is an anti-IgE monoclonal antibody. This treatment has shown to be useful for cases of CRSwNP, asthma, and chronic urticaria. Evidence has shown improvement in objective asthma scores as well as sinonasal symptom scores after 6 months of treatment in patients with allergic asthma and CRSwNP.[63] Mepolizumab is an anti-IL-5 antibody and has been used in the treatment of asthma and eosinophilic granulomatosis with polyangiitis.[1] Studies have shown improvements in asthma exacerbations, SNOT-22 scores, nasal polyp scores, symptoms scores, and blood eosinophils in patients with asthma and CRSwNP.[63]

SUMMARY

There is a close relationship between allergy and certain subtypes of CRSwNP and asthma. When these entities are comorbid, upper and lower airway symptoms are typically caused by type 2 inflammation. Within certain subtypes of CRSwNP, including AFRS, AERD, and CCAD, it is important to recognize the variable prevalence of these comorbid conditions. Further study of the relationship between these disease processes is needed to further improve long-term treatment outcomes for patients.

CLINICS CARE POINTS

- Common therapies include topical corticosteroids, nasal saline irrigations, and ESS for CRSwNP and subtypes of AERD, AFRS, and CCAD; intranasal corticosteroids and oral/topical antihistamines for AR; and inhaled corticosteroids and bronchodilators for asthma.
- When symptoms cannot be controlled with typical therapies, biologic therapies may be an option for patients with CRSwNP and asthma.
- In certain subtypes of disease like AERD, other disease-modifying treatments like aspirin desensitization may be an option.

DISCLOSURES

K G. Bolk: None. T S. Edwards: Research Funding–Sanofi, United States, Regeneron, United States. J M. DelGaudio: Consultant–Medtronic; S K. Wise: Advisory board–Optinose; Consultant–NeurENT, Chitogel, SoundHealth.

REFERENCES

1. Laidlaw TM, Mullol J, Woessner KM, et al. Chronic rhinosinusitis with nasal polyps and asthma. J Allergy Clin Immunol Pract 2021;9(3):1133–41.
2. Anand VK. Epidemiology and economic impact of rhinosinusitis. Ann Otol Rhinol Laryngol 2004;113(5_suppl):3–5.
3. DeConde AS, Soler ZM. Chronic rhinosinusitis: epidemiology and burden of disease. American Journal Of Rhinology & Allergy 2016;30(2):134–9.
4. Steehler AJ, Vuncannon JR, Wise SK, et al. Central compartment atopic disease: outcomes compared with other subtypes of chronic rhinosinusitis with nasal polyps. International Forum Of Allergy & Rhinology 2021;11(11):1549–56.
5. Edwards TS, DelGaudio JM, Levy JM, et al. A Prospective Analysis of Systemic and Local Aeroallergen Sensitivity in Central Compartment Atopic Disease. Otolaryngology-Head Neck Surg (Tokyo) 2022;167(5):885–90.
6. Marcus S, Schertzer J, Roland LT, et al. Central compartment atopic disease: prevalence of allergy and asthma compared with other subtypes of chronic rhinosinusitis with nasal polyps. International Forum Of Allergy & Rhinology 2020;10(2):183–9.
7. Helman SN, Barrow E, Edwards T, et al. The role of allergic rhinitis in chronic rhinosinusitis. Immunol Allergy Clin 2020;40(2):201–14.
8. Husain Q, Sedaghat AR. Understanding and clinical relevance of chronic rhinosinusitis endotypes. Clin Otolaryngol 2019;44(6):887–97.
9. Yip J, Monteiro E, Chan Y. Endotypes of chronic rhinosinusitis. Curr Opin Otolaryngol Head Neck Surg 2019;27(1):14–9.
10. Wilson KF, McMains KC, Orlandi RR. The association between allergy and chronic rhinosinusitis with and without nasal polyps: an evidence-based review with recommendations. International Forum Of Allergy & Rhinology. 2014;4(2):93–103.
11. Orlandi RR, Kingdom TT, Smith TL, et al. International consensus statement on allergy and rhinology: rhinosinusitis 2021. International Forum Of Allergy & Rhinology 2021;11(3):213–739.
12. Murrison LB, Brandt EB, Myers JB, et al. Environmental exposures and mechanisms in allergy and asthma development. J Clin Invest 2019;129(4):1504–15.

13. Wise SK, Damask C, Roland LT, et al. International consensus statement on allergy and rhinology: Allergic rhinitis – 2023. International Forum Of Allergy & Rhinology 2023;13(4):293–859.
14. Gibson PGP, McDonald VMBN, Marks GBP. Asthma in older adults. Lancet (British edition) 2010;376(9743):803–13.
15. Gans MD, Gavrilova T. Understanding the immunology of asthma: pathophysiology, biomarkers, and treatments for asthma endotypes. Paediatric respiratory reviews 2020;36:118–27.
16. Kuruvilla ME, Lee FE-H, Lee GB. Understanding asthma phenotypes, endotypes, and mechanisms of disease. Clin Rev Allergy Immunol 2019;56(2):219–33.
17. Dhami S, Kakourou A, Asamoah F, et al. Allergen immunotherapy for allergic asthma: A systematic review and meta-analysis. Allergy (Cph) 2017;72(12):1825–48.
18. Svenningsen S, Nair P. Asthma endotypes and an overview of targeted therapy for asthma. Front Med 2017;4:158.
19. Kim DK, Eun KM, Kim MK, et al. Comparison between signature cytokines of nasal tissues in subtypes of chronic rhinosinusitis. Allergy, Asthma & Immunology Research 2019;11(2):201–11.
20. Promsopa C, Kansara S, Citardi MJ, et al. Prevalence of confirmed asthma varies in chronic rhinosinusitis subtypes. International Forum Of Allergy & Rhinology 2016;6(4):373–7.
21. Toppila-Salmi S, Hällfors J, Aakko J, et al. The burden of chronic rhinosinusitis with nasal polyps and its relation to asthma in Finland. Clin Transl Allergy 2022;12(10):e12200.
22. Khan AH, Gouia I, Kamat S, et al. Prevalence and severity distribution of type 2 inflammation-related comorbidities among patients with asthma, chronic rhinosinusitis with nasal polyps, and atopic dermatitis. Lung 2023;201(1):57–63.
23. Spector SL, Bernstein IL, Schuller DE, et al. Parameters for the diagnosis and management of sinusitis. Journal of Allergy And Clinical Immunology 1998;102(6):S107–44.
24. Hamada K, Oishi K, Chikumoto A, et al. Impact of sinus surgery on type 2 airway and systemic inflammation in asthma. J Asthma 2021;58(6):750–8.
25. Kennedy JL, Borish L. Chronic sinusitis pathophysiology: the role of allergy. American Journal Of Rhinology & Allergy 2013;27(5):367–71.
26. Fokkens WJ, Hopkins C, Hellings PW, et al. European position paper on rhinosinusitis and nasal polyps 2020. Rhinology 2020;58(Suppl S29):1.
27. Abdullah B, Vengathajalam S, Md Daud MK, et al. The clinical and radiological characterizations of the allergic phenotype of chronic rhinosinusitis with nasal polyps. J Asthma Allergy 2020;13:523–31.
28. Craig TJ. Aeroallergen sensitization in asthma: Prevalence and correlation with severity. Allergy Asthma Proc 2010;31(2):96–102.
29. Proimos E, Papadakis CE, Chimona TS, et al. The effect of functional endoscopic sinus surgery on patients with asthma and CRS with nasal polyps. Rhinology 2010;48(3):331.
30. Kurokawa R, Kanemitsu Y, Fukumitsu K, et al. Nasal polyp eosinophilia and FeNO may predict asthma symptoms development after endoscopic sinus surgery in CRS patients without asthma. J Asthma 2022;59(6):1139–47.
31. Birs I, Boulay ME, Bertrand M, et al. Heterogeneity of asthma with nasal polyposis phenotypes: A cluster analysis. Clin Exp Allergy 2023;53(1):52–64.

32. Won H-K, Kim Y-C, Kang M-G, et al. Age-related prevalence of chronic rhinosinusitis and nasal polyps and their relationships with asthma onset. Ann Allergy Asthma Immunol 2018;120(4):389–94.

33. Lee RU, Stevenson DD. Aspirin-exacerbated respiratory disease: evaluation and management. Allergy, Asthma & Immunology Research 2011;3(1):3–10.

34. Choi J-H, Kim M-A, Park H-S. An update on the pathogenesis of the upper airways in aspirin-exacerbated respiratory disease. Curr Opin Allergy Clin Immunol 2014;14(1):1–6.

35. Nowińska B, Piotrowski J, Dorobisz K. Samter's Triad: pathogenesis, clinical picture, diagnosis, comparison of biological and surgical treatment and the role of aspirin desensitisation. Fam Med Prim Care Rev 2022;24(4):370–4.

36. Laidlaw TM, Boyce JA. Updates on immune mechanisms in aspirin-exacerbated respiratory disease. J Allergy Clin Immunol 2023;151(2):301–9.

37. Levy JM, Rudmik L, Peters AT, et al. Contemporary management of chronic rhinosinusitis with nasal polyposis in aspirin-exacerbated respiratory disease: an evidence-based review with recommendations. International Forum Of Allergy & Rhinology. 2016;6(12):1273–83.

38. DelGaudio JM, Levy JM, Wise SK. Central compartment involvement in aspirin-exacerbated respiratory disease: the role of allergy and previous sinus surgery. International Forum Of Allergy & Rhinology 2019;9(9):1017–22.

39. Bochenek GMDP, Kuschill-Dziurda JMD, Szafraniec KP, et al. Certain subphenotypes of aspirin-exacerbated respiratory disease distinguished by latent class analysis. Journal of Allergy And Clinical Immunology 2014;133(1):98–103.e106.

40. Berges-Gimeno MP, Simon RA, Stevenson DD. The natural history and clinical characteristics of aspirin-exacerbated respiratory disease. Ann Allergy Asthma Immunol 2002;89(5):474–8.

41. Jakiela B, Soja J, Sladek K, et al. Heterogeneity of lower airway inflammation in patients with NSAID-exacerbated respiratory disease. Journal of Allergy And Clinical Immunology 2021;147(4):1269–80.

42. Doña I, Barrionuevo E, Salas M, et al. NSAIDs-hypersensitivity often induces a blended reaction pattern involving multiple organs. Sci Rep 2018;8(1):16710–9.

43. Kato A, Peters AT, Stevens WW, et al. Endotypes of chronic rhinosinusitis: Relationships to disease phenotypes, pathogenesis, clinical findings, and treatment approaches. Allergy (Cph) 2022;77(3):812–26.

44. Buchheit KM, Laidlaw TM. Update on the management of aspirin-exacerbated respiratory disease. Allergy, Asthma & Immunology Research 2016;8(4):298–304.

45. Laidlaw TM, Chu DK, Stevens WW, et al. Controversies in allergy: aspirin desensitization or biologics for aspirin-exacerbated respiratory disease—how to choose. J Allergy Clin Immunol Pract 2022;10(6):1462–7.

46. Mehta MP, Wise SK. Unified airway disease: examining prevalence and treatment of upper airway eosinophilic disease with comorbid asthma. Otolaryngol Clin 2023;56(1):65–81.

47. Laidlaw TM, Mullol J, Fan C, et al. Dupilumab improves nasal polyp burden and asthma control in patients with CRSwNP and AERD. J Allergy Clin Immunol Pract 2019;7(7):2462–5.e2461.

48. Mullur J, Steger CM, Gakpo D, et al. Aspirin desensitization and biologics in aspirin-exacerbated respiratory disease: Efficacy, tolerability, and patient experience. Ann Allergy Asthma Immunol 2022;128(5):575–82.

49. Mullur J, Buchheit KM. Aspirin-exacerbated respiratory disease: Updates in the era of biologics. Ann Allergy Asthma Immunol 2023;131(3):317–24.

50. Bent rJP, Kuhn FA. Diagnosis of allergic fungal sinusitis. Otolaryngology-Head Neck Surg (Tokyo) 1994;111(5):580–8.
51. deShazo RD, Swain RE. Diagnostic criteria for allergic fungal sinusitis. Journal of Allergy And Clinical Immunology 1995;96(1):24–35.
52. Xu T, Guo XT, Zhou YC, et al. Consideration of the Clinical Diagnosis of Allergic Fungal Sinusitis: A Single-Center Retrospective Study. Ear Nose Throat J 2023. https://doi.org/10.1177/01455613231167247. 1455613231167247.
53. Hoyt AEWMD, Borish LMD, Gurrola JMD, et al. Allergic fungal rhinosinusitis. J Allergy Clin Immunol Pract 2016;4(4):599–604.
54. DelGaudio JM. Central compartment atopic disease: the missing link in the allergy and chronic rhinosinusitis with nasal polyps saga. International Forum Of Allergy & Rhinology 2020;10(10):1191–2.
55. Luong A, Davis LS, Marple BF. Peripheral blood mononuclear cells from allergic fungal rhinosinusitis adults express a Th2 cytokine response to fungal antigens. American Journal Of Rhinology & Allergy 2009;23(3):281–7.
56. Millien VO, Lu W, Shaw J, et al. Cleavage of fibrinogen by proteinases elicits allergic responses through toll-like receptor 4. Science (American Association for the Advancement of Science) 2013;341(6147):792–6.
57. Mabry RL, Manning SC, Mabry CS. Immunotherapy in the treatment of allergic fungal sinusitis. Otolaryngology-Head And Neck Surgery 1997;116(1):31–5.
58. Mabry RL, Mabry CS. Immunotherapy for allergic fungal sinusitis: the second year. Otolaryngology-head and Neck Surgery 1997;117(4):367–71.
59. Mabry RL, Marple BF, Folker RJ, et al. Immunotherapy for allergic fungal sinusitis: three years' experience. Otolaryngology-Head Neck Surg (Tokyo) 1998;119(6):648–51.
60. Mabry RL, Marple BF, Mabry CS. Outcomes after discontinuing immunotherapy for allergic fungal sinusitis. Otolaryngology-Head Neck Surg (Tokyo) 2000;122(1):104–6.
61. Doellman MS, Dion GR, Weitzel EK, et al. Immunotherapy in allergic fungal sinusitis: the controversy continues. A recent review of literature. Allergy & Rhinology (Providence, RI) 2013;4(1):e32–5.
62. Lee K, Kim TH, Lee SH, et al. predictive value of radiologic central compartment atopic disease for identifying allergy and asthma in pediatric patients. Ear Nose Throat J 2022;101(9):593–9.
63. Bakakos A, Schleich F, Bakakos P. biological therapy of severe asthma and nasal polyps. J Personalized Med 2022;12(6):976.

Management of Aspirin-Exacerbated Respiratory Disease: What Does the Future Hold?

Erin K. O'Brien, MD[a],*, Elina Jerschow, MD, MSc[b],
Rohit D. Divekar, MBBS, PhD[b]

KEYWORDS

- Aspirin-exacerbated respiratory disease • AERD • Biologic • Arachidonic acid

KEY POINTS

- Aspirin-exacerbated respiratory disease (AERD) is a severe subtype of eosinophilic chronic rhinosinusitis with polyps and asthma with alterations in the arachidonic acid metabolism pathway, characterized by upper and lower airway symptoms after ingestion of aspirin or nonsteroidal anti-inflammatory drugs (NSAIDs).
- Diagnosis of AERD requires a detailed history of aspirin or NSAID ingestion with upper and lower airway reactions, a review of medications for asthma or nasal polyps that may mask aspirin reactions, or an aspirin challenge for those patients with chronic rhinosinusitis with polyps and aspirin without a clear history of aspirin/NSAID reactions.
- Subendotyping within AERD by biomarkers could be useful in the future in selecting appropriate treatment including medications such as aspirin, leukotriene modifiers, or biologics, targeting the altered immune and arachidonic acid metabolism pathways.

INTRODUCTION, HISTORY, DEFINITIONS, BACKGROUND

Aspirin-exacerbated respiratory disease (AERD) is a subtype of chronic rhinosinusitis with polyps (CRSwNP) with asthma and upper and/or lower airway reactions after ingestion of aspirin or nonsteroidal anti-inflammatory drugs (NSAIDs) that inhibit cyclooxygenase 1 (COX-1). This triad is also known as NSAID-exacerbated respiratory disease or Samter's triad after the physician who published a case series in 1968.[1–3] Patients with AERD have recalcitrant nasal polyps and severe asthma and are more likely to have repeated endoscopic sinus surgery for recurrent nasal polyps.[4–8]

---

[a] Department of Otolaryngology–Head and Neck Surgery, Mayo Clinic, Rochester, MN, USA;
[b] Division of Allergic Diseases, Department of Medicine, Mayo Clinic, Rochester, MN, USA
* Corresponding author. Mayo Clinic, 200 First Street Southwest, Rochester, MN 55905.
E-mail address: obrien.erin@mayo.edu

Otolaryngol Clin N Am 57 (2024) 265–278
https://doi.org/10.1016/j.otc.2023.09.006
oto.theclinics.com

INCIDENCE/PREVALENCE

The likelihood of AERD in patients with CRSwNP without asthma is 10% to 16%; in patients with CRSwNP plus asthma is 30% to 40%; and in CRSwNP and severe asthma is estimated at 78%.[3,9–11]

Timing of the onset of symptoms varies, with adult-onset asthma (average age 29 years; 22% as teenagers), then CRSwNP and diminished smell (average age 33 years), and finally reaction to aspirin or NSAIDs.[12] The timing of aspirin reaction could come before polyps are diagnosed (one-quarter of patients), within a year of polyp diagnosis (half), or more than a year after polyps are identified (one-quarter).[12]

DIAGNOSIS
Aspirin Reactions

History of upper or lower airway reactions after ingesting aspirin or NSAIDs is sufficient to diagnose AERD in patients with nasal polyps and asthma.[11,13] Patients should be asked directly about upper airway, lower airway, and gastrointestinal or dermatologic symptoms after taking aspirin or NSAIDs.[11] Up to 75% of patients with AERD may also have airway reactions when drinking alcoholic beverages.[14]

Recognition and diagnosis of AERD can be challenging if a patient has not recently taken aspirin or an NSAID, has delayed development of sensitivity to aspirin, or takes medications that may mask aspirin reactions (**Table 1**).[12,15–18] Recent endoscopic sinus surgery with removal of polyps and inflamed tissue also reduces the likelihood of reaction during an aspirin challenge.[19] Aspirin challenge for diagnosis of AERD should be conducted before sinus surgery if the history of reaction is unclear.[13,15]

Increased awareness of AERD by health care professionals and patients and increased screening of patients with CRSwNP and asthma may decrease the time to diagnosis and improve management of future patients.

Aspirin Challenge

Although a history of aspirin reaction is the standard for diagnosis in patients who had reactions before presenting to doctor's office, the diagnosis can also be made with an aspirin challenge, in which a patient is given doses of aspirin or NSAID in a health care setting to monitor for airway reactions. Increased nasal symptoms or a drop in forced expiratory volume in one second (FEV1) is a positive reaction, confirming the diagnosis of AERD. A negative history of aspirin reaction is insufficient to rule out AERD in patients with nasal polyps and asthma. In a study of aspirin-induced asthma, 15% to 27% of patients with asthma or nasal polyps who were diagnosed

Table 1
Diagnosis of aspirin-exacerbated respiratory disease

Diagnostic Criteria for AERD	Specifics for criteria
History of aspirin reactions to COX-1 inhibitors	Upper airway rhinorrhea, congestion, or sneezing Lower airway wheezing, cough, or asthma exacerbation Gastrointestinal symptoms or rash
Review of recent medications or procedures that may mask a reaction to COX-1 inhibitors	Low-dose daily aspirin Leukotriene-modifying medications Biologics for asthma or nasal polyps Recent endoscopic sinus surgery
Aspirin challenge	Upper and/or lower airway symptoms, drop in FEV1; increased urinary LTE4

with AERD by a positive aspirin challenge were unaware of their aspirin sensitivity.[20,21] A systematic review found 21% of patients with asthma react to aspirin, although prevalence of reported aspirin sensitivity was lower when determined by history than by provocation testing and even lower in medical record review than by prospective patient questionnaires of aspirin/NSAID reactions.[22]

In the future, objective criteria (rather than patient-reported symptoms) could be defined to diagnose a positive aspirin reaction more accurately during a challenge, such as changes in nasal airflow with rhinomanometry, lower airway respiratory changes by spirometry, or acute alterations in systemic or local biomarkers. The development of models for predicting the likelihood of an aspirin reaction and the diagnosis of AERD using clinical data such as the age of onset of disease, the severity of sinus disease, and asthma plus biomarkers from serum, urine, or nasal secretions could obviate the need for aspirin challenges in the future.

Pathophysiology and Biomarkers of Aspirin-Exacerbated Respiratory Disease

AERD is characterized by alterations in arachidonic acid metabolite production and responsiveness. Arachidonic acid is converted to prostaglandins and thromboxanes through the COX pathway or leukotrienes through the 5-lipoxygenase (5-LO) pathway (**Fig. 1**). In AERD, ingestion of COX-1 inhibitors decreases anti-inflammatory prostaglandins and increases pro-inflammatory leukotrienes resulting in nasal congestion, mucus production, and asthma exacerbation with reduced FEV1. However, upper and lower airway symptoms are present even without ingesting COX inhibitors. Subjects with AERD have lower levels of prostaglandin E2, which stabilizes mast cells, and lower prostaglandin E2 (PGE2) receptors and higher pro-inflammatory prostaglandin D2 and cysteinyl leukotrienes (cysLT), as reviewed by Parker and colleagues.[23] The 15-LO, expressed in eosinophils and epithelial and mast cells, is increased in AERD

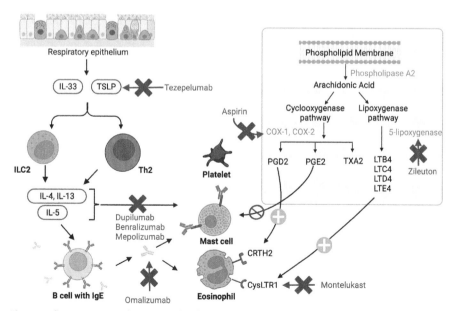

Fig. 1. Inflammatory pathways involved in AERD pathophysiology and potential biomarkers for disease, including inflammatory cytokines and receptors and arachidonic acid metabolites. (Image Created with BioRender.com.)

and induced by interleukin (IL)-4 and IL-13.[24,25] Higher levels of tissue immunoglobulin E (IgE) and IL-5 receptors in AERD indicate a role for these mediators in inflammatory dysregulation.[26] Eosinophils, platelets, innate lymphoid cell type 2 (ILC2), and mast cells are all involved in type 2 inflammation in AERD, with activation by PGD2, leukotrienes, IL-33, and thymic stromal lymphopoietin (TSLP).[27]

Urinary leukotriene E4 (uLTE4), the stable metabolite in the leukotriene pathway, is elevated in patients with AERD.[28] uLTE4 increases after aspirin challenge, and elevated uLTE4 is associated with disease severity and can differentiate AERD from aspirin-tolerant CRSwNP and asthma.[29–31] Urinary leukotriene E4 (LTE4) is currently available through clinical testing as a biomarker for patients with suspected AERD. Further development of urinary LTE4 and additional biomarkers for AERD diagnosis is highly desirable as there is no laboratory test for AERD diagnosis at this time.[32]

Treatment of Aspirin-Exacerbated Respiratory Disease

As there are no AERD-specific therapy options at this time, the current treatment includes management of upper and lower airway symptoms with appropriate treatment for CRSwNP including topical nasal steroids as well as management of asthma, as outlined in clinical practice guidelines.[33–35]

Endoscopic Sinus Surgery

Endoscopic sinus surgery with removal of polyps and inflamed sinonasal tissue in the management of AERD relieves nasal symptoms but also can improve asthma symptoms, increase aspirin tolerance, and decrease systemic inflammation. As reviewed by Muhonen and colleagues, complete endoscopic sinus surgery with bilateral maxillary antrostomies, total ethmoidectomies, sphenoidotomies, and frontal sinusotomies is effective for AERD at improving quality of life, nasal polyp, and sinus radiographic scores.[36] Surgery to remove inflamed tissue decreases systemic LTE4 and prostaglandin D2 (PGD2).[19] Postoperative medical therapy is required to decrease the high recurrence rate of polyps, including topical nasal steroids and aspirin desensitization. Other therapies including leukotriene modifiers and biologics may further reduce polyp recurrence or improve symptoms. One study to date has documented that patients who had endoscopic sinus surgery while on a biologic (dupilumab or benralizumab) for CRSwNP had a greater and sustained improvement in nasal polyp scores compared with patients on biologics alone.[37] The role of biologics plus endoscopic sinus surgery and also potentially in conjunction with aspirin desensitization for patients with AERD should be a focus of future research.

Aspirin Desensitization

Although COX-1 ingestion is associated with acute upper and lower airway reactions in AERD, daily high-dose aspirin intake (325–1300 mg/day) after aspirin challenge and desensitization (aspirin therapy after desensitization [ATAD]) is associated with decreased nasal polyp regrowth and improvement in symptoms after endoscopic sinus surgery.[38] Higher doses of aspirin block COX-2 and COX-1; daily 81 mg aspirin, which blocks only COX-1, does not provide clinical benefit for AERD but may mask reactions during diagnostic aspirin challenge.

Aspirin challenge initially increases PGD2 and LTE4, but after 8 weeks of aspirin, PGD2 decreases without a change in LTE4 or eosinophil levels.[39] ATAD also decreases cysteinyl leukotriene receptor cysLT1 on inflammatory cells, which may explain improved symptoms without a decrease in leukotriene levels, and lowers IL-5.[40,41]

A systematic review and meta-analysis of aspirin desensitization for AERD found ATAD improved overall quality of life, Sino-Nasal Outcome Test (SNOT-22), and respiratory symptoms, but with increased adverse events, including bleeding, gastritis, asthma exacerbation, and rash and need to discontinue aspirin therapy; the effect of aspirin on asthma control was of low certainty.[42]

A survey of patients on ATAD for AERD found 62% still on aspirin therapy for an average of 10 years, whereas 38% had stopped aspirin because of adverse reactions, lack of benefit, or for surgical procedures.[43] Of those still on aspirin, 68% reported no additional sinus surgeries (compared with only 21% of those who stopped aspirin) and increased ability to tolerate drinking alcohol.[43] For patients on ATAD 6 months after endoscopic sinus surgery, one study found few needed escalation of therapy to biologics.[38] Predicting the likelihood of benefit to aspirin therapy for AERD will likely include both clinical variables and biomarkers such as arachidonic acid metabolite and cytokine levels.[44,45]

BIOLOGICS FOR MANAGEMENT OF ASPIRIN-EXACERBATED RESPIRATORY DISEASE

Since 2019, monoclonal antibody therapies (biologics) have been approved for the treatment of CRSwNP, including dupilumab (IL-4 receptor alpha subunit antagonist), mepolizumab (IL-5 inhibitor), and omalizumab (IgE inhibitor). All are also approved for the management of asthma. In addition, tezepelumab (TLSP inhibitor), another biologic currently approved for asthma, is being trialed for CRSwNP management (https://classic.clinicaltrials.gov/ct2/show/NCT04851964). Both benralizumab (IL-5 receptor alpha [IL-5Rα] antibody) (https://classic.clinicaltrials.gov/ct2/show/NCT04157335) and etokimab (anti-IL-33 antibody) (https://clinicaltrials.gov/study/NCT03614923) failed to reach clinically significant improvement in nasal polyp scores and sinonasal symptoms in initial trials in patients with CRSwNP.

In the studies of these biologics for CRSwNP, several included patients with AERD. In the phase 2a trial of dupilumab for CRSwNP, patients with AERD in the treatment arm had a significant reduction in the nasal polyp scores, whereas aspirin-tolerant subjects had a nonstatistically significant reduction in polyp size.[46,47] Additional dupilumab trials found similar improvement in nasal polyp scores between AERD and aspirin-tolerant patients but greater improvements in nasal congestion and SNOT-22 scores in the AERD subjects.[48] As reviewed by Laidlaw and colleagues, in trials for omalizumab and mepolizumab for CRSwNP, subjects with AERD had similar outcomes compared with aspirin-tolerant subjects.[49]

Although there are no direct head-to-head comparisons of biologics for management of AERD, retrospective reviews have found a higher likelihood of AERD patients switching to dupilumab after lack of clinical improvement while on anti-IL-5, IL-5R, or IgE biologics; higher IgE levels were associated with improvement on dupilumab after failure on mepolizumab.[50,51] Dupilumab can decrease urinary LTE4 and increase anti-inflammatory nasal PGE2 in patients with AERD, potentially due to blockage of both IL-4 and IL-13.[52,53] The increase in anti-inflammatory PGE2 may prevent synthesis of pro-inflammatory leukotrienes.

Experimental therapeutics, which is undergoing clinical trials in asthma, may be suitable candidates for future trials in AERD.

Anti-ST2, astegolimab, which targets the IL-33 pathway, has shown some promise in clinical trials for asthma. IL-33 is a pro-inflammatory cytokine that is thought to play a role in the development of airway inflammation and is an alarmin.[54]

Itepekimab, a human IgG4P monoclonal antibody against IL-33, is currently in clinical trials for asthma. Anti-IL-23 risankizumab has also been studied in moderate to severe asthma. IL-23 promotes Th17-cell proliferation, neutrophil recruitment, and Th2 cytokine production.

These are just a few of the experimental therapeutics that are being investigated for the treatment of AERD. As more research is conducted, it is possible that other promising treatments will be identified.

BIOLOGICS TO IMPROVE ASPIRIN TOLERANCE

Biologics can reduce the severity of airway reactions during aspirin challenge in patients with AERD.[55] Patients with AERD treated with a biologic for asthma for 6 months had a complete or higher tolerance to aspirin during a challenge including benralizumab (4/9 patients); dupilumab (6/10), mepolizumab (3/9), or omalizumab (9/10).[55] Other studies of omalizumab similarly found complete or higher tolerance to aspirin challenge in a majority of patients, possibly through suppression of LTE4 and PGD2 production, but reactions can still occur on omalizumab.[56–60] Although mepolizumab can also decrease LTE4 and PGD2 production, it does not consistently prevent aspirin reactions.[61,62]

Dupilumab can also increase tolerance to aspirin in AERD subjects during aspirin challenge.[18] Of 30 AERD patients treated with dupilumab for 6 months, 7 had complete aspirin tolerance, and 10 tolerated a higher dose of aspirin (57% total), with increased tolerance associated with decreased urinary LTE4 levels.[18] The aspirin-intolerant patients had higher disease burden.[18]

There are no current data on comparisons of biologics for AERD, on the role of biologics in combination with other therapies such as aspirin after desensitization or leukotriene modifying medications, nor for preventing polyp recurrence after endoscopic sinus surgery. As AERD often requires multimodality therapy, the selection and combination of therapies with biologics as well as the duration of biologic therapy will be an important area of study. As new biologics are trialed for management of CRSwNP, including tezepelumab, the outcomes for AERD subjects and changes in biomarkers associated with AERD should be specifically examined and reported.

LEUKOTRIENE-MODIFYING MEDICATIONS

Overproduction and increased reactivity to leukotrienes in AERD can be targeted with medications to block leukotriene receptors or leukotriene production. Montelukast and zafirlukast block cysteinyl leukotriene receptor cysLTR1, located on eosinophils and pulmonary smooth muscle cells, but not cysLTR2 or cysLTR3 (GPR99) receptors.[63,64] Zileuton inhibits 5-lipoxygenase, which converts arachidonic acid to leukotrienes with a decrease in LTE4, as reviewed by Berger and colleagues.[65]

Leukotriene-modifying medications may decrease reactions during aspirin desensitization. However, higher tryptase levels were associated with reduced effectiveness of montelukast, possibly through activation of mast cells by receptors other than cysLTR1. In contrast, zileuton blocked both aspirin reactions and the increases in LTE4 and tryptase levels during aspirin challenge.[16,66,67] Increased effectiveness of zileuton at blocking aspirin reactions may also be due to cysLTR2 receptors in the upper airway, not inhibited by montelukast.[68]

Leukotriene modifiers for management of AERD may improve asthma and nasal symptoms and airflow with montelukast and zileuton, although benefit was limited in some studies.[69–71] In a review of patients with AERD treated with montelukast and budesonide sinus rinses, 19 of 40 patients were switched to zileuton, with some improvement in SNOT-22 symptoms and endoscopy scores.[72] Treatment with zileuton after endoscopic sinus surgery in AERD patients did not decrease antibiotic or steroid use, sinusitis exacerbations, or sinus symptom scores but decreased the need for revision endoscopic sinus surgery.[71] Despite evidence of benefit of zileuton, in a survey of patients with AERD, only 24% had ever been on zileuton; 43% of those who tried it stopped because it was ineffective, whereas 28% found it highly effective.[73]

Using leukotriene modifiers in combination with aspirin therapy or biologics or targeting additional leukotriene receptors are potential targets for AERD research.

EOSINOPHILS AND MAST CELLS

Patients with AERD have higher serum and tissue eosinophils and mast cells. Targeting these cells directly could improve AERD management, although some studies have not shown significant benefits.

In a trial targeting eosinophils, 16 patients with CRSwNP and asthma (three with AERD) were treated with dexpramipexole to decrease eosinophils. After 6 months, there was no significant improvement in nasal polyp scores, SNOT-22 or olfactory testing scores, or asthma control.[74] As IL-5 antagonist mepolizumab had no significant difference in improvement in AERD subjects compared with aspirin-tolerant CRSwNP, it is unlikely that reducing eosinophilic inflammation alone is sufficient to control symptoms in AERD.[49]

As reviewed by Boyce, medications targeting mast cells are another avenue for research in AERD, including blockage of mast cell activators IL-33 or TSLP.[75] Mast cell stabilizer cromolyn can decrease asthma reactions and LTE4 levels with aspirin challenge but no reports regarding effects on nasal symptoms with AERD.[76,77]

Patients with AERD have higher pro-inflammatory PGD2, which is released from mast cells and binds to eosinophils, ILC2 and Th2 cells, and basophils via the chemo-attractant receptor-homologous molecule expressed on T-helper type 2 cells (CRTH2) receptor.[78] In a trial of CRTH2 antagonist AZD1981, 22 subjects with CRSwNP (13 with AERD) treated for 12 weeks had no significant improvement in nasal polyp scores, Lund Mackay CT scan scores, SNOT-22, or smell test scores or inflammatory markers.[78] A trial of CRTH2 antagonist fevipiprant for CRSwNP with comorbid asthma found no benefit in nasal polyps reduction, SNOT-22 symptoms, or smell test scores; only one subject had AERD.[79] Blockade of PGD2 alone does not seem to affect disease in CRSwNP or AERD.

PLATELETS

Platelet activation and adherence to leukocytes may play a role in aspirin reaction and disease in AERD. To test the effect of blockage of platelet activation on aspirin reactions, 40 patients were treated with prasugrel, a P2Y12 platelet activation receptor antagonist or placebo in a crossover study with aspirin challenges.[80] Thirty-five subjects did not have a change in nasal symptoms, number of platelet-leukocyte aggregates, or increases in LTE4 and PGD2, and only five patients had no reaction to the aspirin challenge while on prasugrel, indicating only a small subset of AERD patients had P2y12 platelet-mediated reactions to aspirin.[80]

As pro-inflammatory prostaglandins and thromboxanes are implicated in AERD, a thromboxane-prostanoid receptor antagonist ifetroban or placebo was given to 35 AERD subjects for 4 weeks before aspirin challenge.[81] The ifetroban group had lower urinary LTE4 but also lower nasal PGE2 and greater increase in nasal symptoms with aspirin challenge and a larger decline in FEV1 than the placebo group. The investigators hypothesized that ifetroban decreased the protective effect of PGE2 in "braking" the aspirin reaction in subjects with AERD.[81]

DIET

Several trials have examined the effect of diet on AERD symptoms. Arachidonic acid from dietary omega-6 fatty acids is converted to pro-inflammatory leukotrienes, prostaglandins, and thromboxanes. Omega-3 fatty acids are metabolized to anti-inflammatory molecules that modulate omega-6 derivatives. Western diets high in omega-6 fatty acids (corn and soybean oil, corn-fed meat, and dairy) and low in omega-3 fatty acid consumption (cold water fish, nuts, and seeds) have elevated ratios of omega-6 to omega-3 in tissue phospholipids.[82] Ten patients with AERD on a low omega-6, high omega-3 diet for 2 weeks had lower urinary LTE4 and PGD2 derivatives, lower SNOT-22 scores, and some improvement in asthma.[83]

Studies of low salicylate diets for AERD found improved sinonasal and asthma symptoms and nasal endoscopy but no change in urinary salicylates or leukotrienes.[84,85] It is unclear if dietary salicylates can affect the COX-1 pathway. Aspirin is acetylated salicylic acid and transfers the acetyl group to a serine on the COX-1 enzyme to irreversibly block the enzyme. As dietary salicylates are not acetylated, it is unlikely these food derivatives that significantly contribute to COX-1 inhibition.[83]

The possible role of diet in AERD pathogenesis and management warrants future research, including measurement of biomarkers with dietary changes.

SUBENDOTYPING: BIOMARKERS TO CHOOSE ASPIRIN-EXACERBATED RESPIRATORY DISEASE THERAPY

AERD has variability in terms of severity of disease and response to treatment. An analysis of inflammatory cytokines from nasal mucus in 30 patients with AERD, compared with 109 patients with CRSwNP without AERD, found higher levels of IL-5, IL-6, IL-13, and interferon-gamma (IFN-γ) in AERD.[86] Hierarchical cluster analysis identified three inflammatory subendotypes in the AERD samples, including a third of AERD with low inflammatory burden; half with high type 2 inflammatory cluster (IL-4, IL-5, and IL-13 as well as high IL-6), and about 20% of subjects with low type 2 inflammation and high type 1 (IFN-γ) and type 3 (IL-17A) inflammation. Patients in cluster 2 with higher type 2 inflammation had the highest eosinophil counts, worse SNOT-22 scores, and were more likely to have severe asthma. Differences in response to aspirin therapy, leukotriene modifiers, and biologics in both reactions to aspirin challenges and improvement in AERD symptoms indicate a need to subendotype AERD patients. Patient symptoms, demographics, and serum or nasal biomarkers could be used to create algorithms for predicting and monitoring the appropriate medical therapies.

SUMMARY

AERD is a severe phenotype of CRSwNP that may require more diligent diagnosis and treatment beyond nasal steroids and endoscopic sinus surgery. Selection of extent of surgery and postoperative systemic therapies including aspirin desensitization and therapy, dietary changes, leukotriene modifiers, biologics, or other medications to block targets in the inflammatory pathway will require additional research in biomarkers for diagnosis, AERD subendotyping, and monitoring of response to therapy.

CLINICS CARE POINTS

- Increased awareness and improved diagnosis of aspirin-exacerbated respiratory disease (AERD) is needed to tailor treatment of more recalcitrant polyp disease and more severe asthma.

- Identification of biomarkers for AERD will aid in diagnosis, choice of therapeutic options, and monitoring of treatment response.
- Biologics approved for asthma or chronic rhinosinusitis with polyps (CRSwNP) should be studied specifically in patients in AERD to identify therapeutic options for this subtype of CRSwNP, including timing of biologic therapy with endoscopic sinus surgery.

DISCLOSURE

Dr E. Jerschow received research funding from Regeneron, United States. The rest of the authors declare that they have no relevant financial relationships.

REFERENCES

1. Samter M, Beers RF Jr. Intolerance to aspirin. Clinical studies and consideration of its pathogenesis. Ann Intern Med 1968;68(5):975–83.
2. Laidlaw TM, Levy JM. NSAID-ERD syndrome: the new hope from prevention, early diagnosis, and new therapeutic targets. Curr Allergy Asthma Rep 2020; 20(4):10.
3. Stevens WW, Peters AT, Hirsch AG, et al. Clinical characteristics of patients with chronic rhinosinusitis with nasal polyps, asthma, and aspirin-exacerbated respiratory disease. J Allergy Clin Immunol Pract 2017;5(4):1061–1070 e1063.
4. Loftus CA, Soler ZM, Koochakzadeh S, et al. Revision surgery rates in chronic rhinosinusitis with nasal polyps: meta-analysis of risk factors. Int Forum Allergy Rhinol 2020;10(2):199–207.
5. Mascia K, Haselkorn T, Deniz YM, et al. Aspirin sensitivity and severity of asthma: Evidence for irreversible airway obstruction in patients with severe or difficult-to-treat asthma. J Allergy Clin Immunol 2005;116(5):970–5.
6. Lee Y, Kim C, Lee E, et al. Long-term clinical outcomes of aspirin-exacerbated respiratory disease: Real-world data from an adult asthma cohort. Clin Exp Allergy 2023;53(9):941–50.
7. Bayer K, Hamidovic S, Besser G, et al. Factors Associated with Revision Sinus Surgery in Patients with Chronic Rhinosinusitis. J Pers Med 2022;12(2).
8. Morales DR, Guthrie B, Lipworth BJ, et al. NSAID-exacerbated respiratory disease: a meta-analysis evaluating prevalence, mean provocative dose of aspirin and increased asthma morbidity. Allergy 2015;70(7):828–35.
9. Kshirsagar RS, Chou DW, Wei J, et al. Aspirin-exacerbated respiratory disease: longitudinal assessment of a large cohort and implications of diagnostic delay. Int Forum Allergy Rhinol 2020;10(4):465–73.
10. Stevenson DD, Szczeklik A. Clinical and pathologic perspectives on aspirin sensitivity and asthma. J Allergy Clin Immunol 2006;118(4):773–86, quiz 787-778.
11. White AA, Stevenson DD. Aspirin-Exacerbated Respiratory Disease. N Engl J Med 2018;379(23):2281–2.
12. Buchheit K, Bensko JC, Lewis E, et al. The importance of timely diagnosis of aspirin-exacerbated respiratory disease for patient health and safety. World J Otorhinolaryngol Head Neck Surg 2020;6(4):203–6.
13. Khan DA, Banerji A, Blumenthal KG, et al. Drug allergy: A 2022 practice parameter update. J Allergy Clin Immunol 2022;150(6):1333–93.
14. Cardet JC, White AA, Barrett NA, et al. Alcohol-induced respiratory symptoms are common in patients with aspirin exacerbated respiratory disease. J Allergy Clin Immunol Pract 2014;2(2):208–13.

15. Stevens WW, Jerschow E, Baptist AP, et al. The role of aspirin desensitization followed by oral aspirin therapy in managing patients with aspirin-exacerbated respiratory disease: a work group report from the rhinitis, rhinosinusitis and ocular allergy committee of the American academy of allergy, asthma & immunology. J Allergy Clin Immunol 2021;147(3):827–44.

16. Israel E, Fischer AR, Rosenberg MA, et al. The pivotal role of 5-lipoxygenase products in the reaction of aspirin-sensitive asthmatics to aspirin. Am Rev Respir Dis 1993;148(6 Pt 1):1447–51.

17. Stevenson DD, Simon RA, Mathison DA, et al. Montelukast is only partially effective in inhibiting aspirin responses in aspirin-sensitive asthmatics. Ann Allergy Asthma Immunol 2000;85(6):477–82.

18. Schneider S, Poglitsch K, Morgenstern C, et al. Dupilumab increases aspirin tolerance in NSAID-exacerbated respiratory disease. Eur Respir J 2023;61(3).

19. Jerschow E, Edin ML, Chi Y, et al. Sinus Surgery Is Associated with a Decrease in Aspirin-Induced Reaction Severity in Patients with Aspirin Exacerbated Respiratory Disease. J Allergy Clin Immunol Pract 2019;7(5):1580–8.

20. Szczeklik A, Nizankowska E, Duplaga M. Natural history of aspirin-induced asthma. AIANE Investigators. European Network on Aspirin-Induced Asthma. Eur Respir J 2000;16(3):432–6.

21. Dages KN, Sofola-James O, Sehanobish E, et al. Sex, Ethnicity, Body Mass Index, and Environmental Exposures Associated With NSAID-Exacerbated Respiratory Disease Symptom Sequence. J Allergy Clin Immunol Pract 2023;S2213-2198(23) 00809-7.

22. Jenkins C, Costello J, Hodge L. Systematic review of prevalence of aspirin induced asthma and its implications for clinical practice. Bmj 2004;328(7437):434.

23. Parker AR, Ayars AG, Altman MC, et al. Lipid mediators in aspirin-exacerbated respiratory disease. Immunol Allergy Clin North Am 2016;36(4):749–63.

24. Chaitidis P, O'Donnell V, Kuban RJ, et al. Gene expression alterations of human peripheral blood monocytes induced by medium-term treatment with the TH2-cytokines interleukin-4 and -13. Cytokine 2005;30(6):366–77.

25. James A, Daham K, Backman L, et al. The influence of aspirin on release of eoxin C4, leukotriene C4 and 15-HETE, in eosinophilic granulocytes isolated from patients with asthma. Int Arch Allergy Immunol 2013;162(2):135–42.

26. Buchheit KM, Dwyer DF, Ordovas-Montanes J, et al. IL-5Ralpha marks nasal polyp IgG4- and IgE-expressing cells in aspirin-exacerbated respiratory disease. J Allergy Clin Immunol 2020;145(6):1574–84.

27. Lyly A, Laidlaw TM, Lundberg M. Pathomechanisms of AERD-Recent Advances. Front Allergy 2021;2:734733.

28. Divekar R, Hagan J, Rank M, et al. Diagnostic Utility of Urinary LTE4 in Asthma, Allergic Rhinitis, Chronic Rhinosinusitis, Nasal Polyps, and Aspirin Sensitivity. J Allergy Clin Immunol Pract 2016;4(4):665–70.

29. Sanak M, Kiełbasa B, Bochenek G, et al. Exhaled eicosanoids following oral aspirin challenge in asthmatic patients. Clin Exp Allergy 2004;34(12):1899–904.

30. Bochenek G, Stachura T, Szafraniec K, et al. Diagnostic Accuracy of Urinary LTE4 Measurement to Predict Aspirin-Exacerbated Respiratory Disease in Patients with Asthma. J Allergy Clin Immunol Pract 2018;6(2):528–35.

31. Hagan JB, Laidlaw TM, Divekar R, et al. Urinary Leukotriene E4 to Determine Aspirin Intolerance in Asthma: A Systematic Review and Meta-Analysis. J Allergy Clin Immunol Pract 2017;5(4):990–997 e991.

32. Rhyou HI, Nam YH, Park HS. Emerging Biomarkers Beyond Leukotrienes for the Management of Nonsteroidal Anti-inflammatory Drug (NSAID)-Exacerbated Respiratory Disease. Allergy Asthma Immunol Res 2022;14(2):153–67.

33. Cloutier MM, Baptist AP, Blake KV, et al. Focused Updates to the Asthma Management Guidelines: A Report from the National Asthma Education and Prevention Program Coordinating Committee Expert Panel Working Group. J Allergy Clin Immunol 2020;146(6):1217–70.

34. Fokkens WJ, Lund VJ, Hopkins C, et al. European Position Paper on Rhinosinusitis and Nasal Polyps 2020. Rhinology 2020;58(Suppl S29):1–464.

35. Orlandi RR, Kingdom TT, Smith TL, et al. International consensus statement on allergy and rhinology: rhinosinusitis 2021. Int Forum Allergy Rhinol 2021;11(3): 213–739.

36. Muhonen EG, Goshtasbi K, Papagiannopoulos P, et al. Appropriate extent of surgery for aspirin-exacerbated respiratory disease. World J Otorhinolaryngol Head Neck Surg 2020;6(4):235–40.

37. Garvey E, Naimi B, Duffy A, et al. Optimizing the timing of biologic and surgical therapy for patients with refractory chronic rhinosinusitis with nasal polyposis (CRSwNP). Int Forum Allergy Rhinol 2023. https://doi.org/10.1002/alr.23246.

38. Sweis AM, Locke TB, Ig-Izevbekhai KI, et al. Effectiveness of endoscopic sinus surgery and aspirin therapy in the management of aspirin-exacerbated respiratory disease. Allergy Asthma Proc 2021;42(2):136–41.

39. Cahill KN, Bensko JC, Boyce JA, et al. Prostaglandin D_2: a dominant mediator of aspirin-exacerbated respiratory disease. J Allergy Clin Immunol 2015;135(1): 245–52.

40. Sousa AR, Parikh A, Scadding G, et al. Leukotriene-Receptor Expression on Nasal Mucosal Inflammatory Cells in Aspirin-Sensitive Rhinosinusitis. N Engl J Med 2002;347(19):1493–9.

41. Mortazavi N, Esmaeilzadeh H, Abbasinazari M, et al. Clinical and Immunological Efficacy of Aspirin Desensitization in Nasal Polyp Patients with Aspirin-Exacerbated Respiratory Disease. Iran J Pharm Res (IJPR) 2017;16(4):1639–47.

42. Chu DK, Lee DJ, Lee KM, et al. Benefits and harms of aspirin desensitization for aspirin-exacerbated respiratory disease: a systematic review and meta-analysis. Int Forum Allergy Rhinol 2019;9(12):1409–19.

43. Walters KM, Waldram JD, Woessner KM, et al. Long-term Clinical Outcomes of Aspirin Desensitization With Continuous Daily Aspirin Therapy in Aspirin-exacerbated Respiratory Disease. Am J Rhinol Allergy 2018;32(4):280–6.

44. Jerschow E, Edin ML, Pelletier T, et al. Plasma 15-Hydroxyeicosatetraenoic Acid Predicts Treatment Outcomes in Aspirin-Exacerbated Respiratory Disease. J Allergy Clin Immunol Pract 2017;5(4):998–1007, e1002.

45. Mastalerz L, Tyrak KE. Biomarkers for predicting response to long-term high dose aspirin therapy in aspirin-exacerbated respiratory disease. Clin Transl Allergy 2021;11(6):e12048.

46. Laidlaw TM, Mullol J, Fan C, et al. Dupilumab improves nasal polyp burden and asthma control in patients with CRSwNP and AERD. J Allergy Clin Immunol Pract 2019;7(7):2462–5.e2461.

47. Bachert C, Mannent L, Naclerio RM, et al. Effect of Subcutaneous Dupilumab on Nasal Polyp Burden in Patients With Chronic Sinusitis and Nasal Polyposis: A Randomized Clinical Trial. JAMA 2016;315(5):469–79.

48. Mullol J, Laidlaw TM, Bachert C, et al. Efficacy and safety of dupilumab in patients with uncontrolled severe chronic rhinosinusitis with nasal polyps and a

clinical diagnosis of NSAID-ERD: Results from two randomized placebo-controlled phase 3 trials. Allergy 2022;77(4):1231–44.

49. Laidlaw TM, Chu DK, Stevens WW, et al. Controversies in Allergy: Aspirin Desensitization or Biologics for Aspirin-Exacerbated Respiratory Disease-How to Choose. J Allergy Clin Immunol Pract 2022;10(6):1462–7.

50. Wangberg H, Spierling Bagsic SR, Osuna L, et al. Appraisal of the Real-World Effectiveness of Biologic Therapies in Aspirin-Exacerbated Respiratory Disease. J Allergy Clin Immunol Pract 2022;10(2):478–84.e473.

51. Bavaro N, Gakpo D, Mittal A, et al. Efficacy of dupilumab in patients with aspirin-exacerbated respiratory disease and previous inadequate response to anti-IL-5 or anti-IL-5Rα in a real-world setting. J Allergy Clin Immunol Pract 2021;9(7):2910–2, e2911.

52. Buchheit KM, Sohail A, Hacker J, et al. Rapid and sustained effect of dupilumab on clinical and mechanistic outcomes in aspirin-exacerbated respiratory disease. J Allergy Clin Immunol 2022;150(2):415–24.

53. Picado C, Mullol J, Roca-Ferrer J. Mechanisms by which dupilumab normalizes eicosanoid metabolism and restores aspirin-tolerance in AERD: A hypothesis. J Allergy Clin Immunol 2023;151(2):310–3.

54. Kelsen SG, Agache IO, Soong W, et al. Astegolimab (anti-ST2) efficacy and safety in adults with severe asthma: A randomized clinical trial. J Allergy Clin Immunol 2021;148(3):790–8.

55. Sánchez J, García E, Lopez JF, et al. Nonsteroidal Anti-inflammatory Drug (NSAID) Tolerance After Biological Therapy in Patients With NSAID-Exacerbated Respiratory Disease: A Randomized Comparative Trial. J Allergy Clin Immunol Pract 2023;11(7):2172–9.

56. Quint T, Dahm V, Ramazanova D, et al. Omalizumab-Induced Aspirin Tolerance in Nonsteroidal Anti-Inflammatory Drug-Exacerbated Respiratory Disease Patients Is Independent of Atopic Sensitization. J Allergy Clin Immunol Pract 2022;10(2):506–16.e506.

57. Lang DM, Aronica MA, Maierson ES, et al. Omalizumab can inhibit respiratory reaction during aspirin desensitization. Ann Allergy Asthma Immunol 2018;121(1):98–104.

58. Waldram J, Walters K, Simon R, et al. Safety and outcomes of aspirin desensitization for aspirin-exacerbated respiratory disease: A single-center study. J Allergy Clin Immunol 2018;141(1):250–6.

59. Hayashi H, Fukutomi Y, Mitsui C, et al. Omalizumab for Aspirin Hypersensitivity and Leukotriene Overproduction in Aspirin-exacerbated Respiratory Disease. A Randomized Controlled Trial. Am J Respir Crit Care Med 2020;201(12):1488–98.

60. Hayashi H, Mitsui C, Nakatani E, et al. Omalizumab reduces cysteinyl leukotriene and 9α,11β-prostaglandin F2 overproduction in aspirin-exacerbated respiratory disease. J Allergy Clin Immunol 2016;137(5):1585–7.e1584.

61. Buchheit KM, Lewis E, Gakpo D, et al. Mepolizumab targets multiple immune cells in aspirin-exacerbated respiratory disease. J Allergy Clin Immunol 2021;148(2):574–84.

62. Martin H, Barrett NA, Laidlaw T. Mepolizumab does not prevent all aspirin-induced reactions in patients with aspirin-exacerbated respiratory disease: A case series. J Allergy Clin Immunol Pract 2021;9(3):1384–5.

63. Kanaoka Y, Maekawa A, Austen KF. Identification of GPR99 Protein as a Potential Third Cysteinyl Leukotriene Receptor with a Preference for Leukotriene E4 Ligand. J Biol Chem 2013;288(16):10967–72.

64. Bankova LG, Lai J, Yoshimoto E, et al. Leukotriene E4 elicits respiratory epithelial cell mucin release through the G-protein-coupled receptor, GPR99. Proc Natl Acad Sci U S A 2016;113(22):6242–7.

65. Berger W, De Chandt MT, Cairns CB. Zileuton: clinical implications of 5-Lipoxygenase inhibition in severe airway disease. Int J Clin Pract 2007;61(4):663–76.

66. Cahill KN, Murphy K, Singer J, et al. Plasma tryptase elevation during aspirin-induced reactions in aspirin-exacerbated respiratory disease. J Allergy Clin Immunol 2019;143(2):799–803.e792.

67. Fischer AR, Rosenberg MA, Lilly CM, et al. Direct evidence for a role of the mast cell in the nasal response to aspirin in aspirin-sensitive asthma. J Allergy Clin Immunol 1994;94(6 Pt 1):1046–56.

68. White A, Ludington E, Mehra P, et al. Effect of leukotriene modifier drugs on the safety of oral aspirin challenges. Ann Allergy Asthma Immunol 2006;97(5):688–93.

69. Dahlén B, Nizankowska E, Szczeklik A, et al. Benefits from adding the 5-lipoxygenase inhibitor zileuton to conventional therapy in aspirin-intolerant asthmatics. Am J Respir Crit Care Med 1998;157(4 Pt 1):1187–94.

70. Micheletto C, Tognella S, Visconti M, et al. Montelukast 10 mg improves nasal function and nasal response to aspirin in ASA-sensitive asthmatics: a controlled study vs placebo. Allergy 2004;59(3):289–94.

71. Lee SE, Farquhar DR, Adams KN, et al. Effect of Zileuton Treatment on Sinonasal Quality of Life in Patients with Aspirin-Exacerbated Respiratory Disease. Am J Rhinol Allergy 2019;33(6):791–5.

72. Makary CA, Holmes T, Unsal A, et al. Long-term role of zileuton in the treatment of chronic rhinosinusitis in aspirin exacerbated respiratory disease. Am J Otolaryngol 2022;43(1):103227.

73. Ta V, White AA. Survey-Defined Patient Experiences With Aspirin-Exacerbated Respiratory Disease. J Allergy Clin Immunol Pract 2015;3(5):711–8.

74. Laidlaw TM, Prussin C, Panettieri RA, et al. Dexpramipexole depletes blood and tissue eosinophils in nasal polyps with no change in polyp size. Laryngoscope 2019;129(2):E61–6.

75. Boyce JA. Aspirin sensitivity: Lessons in the regulation (and dysregulation) of mast cell function. J Allergy Clin Immunol 2019;144(4):875–81.

76. Robuschi M, Gambaro G, Sestini P, et al. Attenuation of aspirin-induced bronchoconstriction by sodium cromoglycate and nedocromil sodium. Am J Respir Crit Care Med 1997;155(4):1461–4.

77. Yoshida S, Amayasu H, Sakamoto H, et al. Cromolyn sodium prevents bronchoconstriction and urinary LTE4 excretion in aspirin-induced asthma. Ann Allergy Asthma Immunol 1998;80(2):171–6.

78. Price CPE, Guo A, Stevens WW, et al. Efficacy of an oral CRTH2 antagonist (AZD1981) in the treatment of chronic rhinosinusitis with nasal polyps in adults: A randomized controlled clinical trial. Clin Exp Allergy 2022;52(7):859–67.

79. Gevaert P, Bachert C, Maspero JF, et al. Phase 3b randomized controlled trial of fevipiprant in patients with nasal polyposis with asthma (THUNDER). J Allergy Clin Immunol 2022;149(5):1675–82.e1673.

80. Laidlaw TM, Cahill KN, Cardet JC, et al. A trial of type 12 purinergic (P2Y(12)) receptor inhibition with prasugrel identifies a potentially distinct endotype of patients with aspirin-exacerbated respiratory disease. J Allergy Clin Immunol 2019;143(1):316–24.e317.

81. Laidlaw TM, Buchheit KM, Cahill KN, et al. Trial of thromboxane receptor inhibition with ifetroban: TP receptors regulate eicosanoid homeostasis in aspirin-exacerbated respiratory disease. J Allergy Clin Immunol 2023;152(3):700–10.e3.

82. Blasbalg TL, Hibbeln JR, Ramsden CE, et al. Changes in consumption of omega-3 and omega-6 fatty acids in the United States during the 20th century. Am J Clin Nutr 2011;93(5):950–62.

83. Schneider TR, Johns CB, Palumbo ML, et al. Dietary Fatty Acid Modification for the Treatment of Aspirin-Exacerbated Respiratory Disease: A Prospective Pilot Trial. J Allergy Clin Immunol Pract 2018;6(3):825–31.

84. Sommer DD, Rotenberg BW, Sowerby LJ, et al. A novel treatment adjunct for aspirin exacerbated respiratory disease: the low-salicylate diet: a multicenter randomized control crossover trial. Int Forum Allergy Rhinol 2016;6(4):385–91.

85. Sowerby LJ, Patel KB, Schmerk C, et al. Effect of low salicylate diet on clinical and inflammatory markers in patients with aspirin exacerbated respiratory disease - a randomized crossover trial. J Otolaryngol Head Neck Surg 2021;50(1):27.

86. Scott WC, Cahill KN, Milne GL, et al. Inflammatory heterogeneity in aspirin-exacerbated respiratory disease. J Allergy Clin Immunol 2021;147(4):1318–28.e1315.

Update on the Role of Fungus in Allergy, Asthma, and the Unified Airway

Brian H. Cameron, MD[a], Shaina W. Gong, MD[a],
David B. Corry, MD[b], Amber U. Luong, MD, PhD[a,c],*

KEYWORDS

- Fungi • Asthma • Rhinosinusitis • Allergic fungal rhinosinusitis • Airway mycosis

KEY POINTS

- Presentation of fungi-mediated airway inflammation in part depends on immune status of the affected host.
- Numerous fungal elements and signaling pathways have recently been described and associated with fungi-mediated airway inflammation.
- Better understanding of the molecular pathophysiology in fungi-mediated respiratory diseases have led to exploring more customized management including earlier sinus surgery with postoperative topical corticosteroids, biologics, and topical antifungals or antimicrobial peptides.

INTRODUCTION

The unified airway refers to the combined upper and lower airways and their shared pathophysiologic relationships. These 2 systems are thought to be interconnected, and disease processes such as asthma, allergic rhinitis (AR), chronic rhinosinusitis (CRS), and chronic otitis media are thought to be linked, requiring an integrated approach to control inflammation throughout the entire airway.[1] Indeed, up to 50% of patients with chronic rhinosinusitis with nasal polyps (CRSwNP) have been found to have coexisting asthma.[2,3] Similarly, 15% and 60% of asthmatics have been shown to have coexisting CRSwNP and AR, respectively.[2] As patients with inflammatory disease in either the upper or lower airways have a high likelihood of concurrent disease in the remaining airway, it is thought these 2 locations function as a single,

[a] Department of Otorhinolaryngology – Head and Neck Surgery, McGovern Medical School at the University of Texas Health Science Center, 6431 Fannin Street, MSB 5.036, Houston, TX, USA; [b] Department of Medicine, Biology of Inflammation Center, Baylor College of Medicine, One Baylor Plaza, Houston, 77030 TX, USA; [c] Center for Immunology and Autoimmune Diseases, Institute of Molecular Medicine, 1835 Pressler, Houston, TX, 77030 USA
* Corresponding author. 6431 Fannin Street, MSB 5.036, Houston, TX 77030.
E-mail address: amber.u.luong@uth.tmc.edu

Otolaryngol Clin N Am 57 (2024) 279–292
https://doi.org/10.1016/j.otc.2023.09.005
0030-6665/24/© 2023 Elsevier Inc. All rights reserved.

integrated unit. In this way, diseases that stimulate inflammation in one portion of the airway are thought to cause similar reactions in the remaining airway.

Diseases affecting the unified airway have processes related to atopy, where a cascade of cytokines is produced in response to specific environmental agents, including fungal organisms. In fact, asthma and CRS are often linked to noninvasive growth of fungi, termed airway mycosis. There are many factors that influence prevalence and pathogenicity of type 2 inflammatory reactions to fungi. In these cases, the influence of geography and climate should not be ignored. Increases in temperature and rainfall can lead to increased mold growth, which has been linked to inflammatory airway conditions such as allergic fungal rhinosinusitis (AFRS), bronchopulmonary aspergillosis, and hypersensitivity pneumonitis.[4] For AFRS, the region with the highest reported prevalence is typically found in the southern United States, which is commonly associated with subtropical and wet equatorial climates.[5] Conversely, regions with moist climates and cold winters such as the northeast United States have significantly fewer cases of AFRS.[6] Because the effects of climate change lead to changing temperatures and weather patterns, it will be important to monitor the resulting changes in fungal exposure and its effects on reactive airway diseases.

Before looking forward to the potential changes that may occur in the geographic distribution of fungal species and their likely effects on reactive airway disease, it is important to examine recent developments in our understanding of the role of fungus in driving the inflammation seen in both upper and lower airway diseases. This review will provide such an update and will discuss future directions for investigation.

FUNCTION OF IMMUNE RESPONSES AND LINKAGE TO INFLAMMATORY RESPIRATORY DISEASES

There are 3 types of innate and adaptive cell-mediated effector immune responses known as type 1, 2, and 3. This diversity of responses provides protection against a variety of pathogenic microorganisms that exist in our environment. Type 1 immunity is associated with autoimmune disease as well as responses to intracellular bacteria, protozoa, and viruses through Type 1 innate lymphoid cells and adaptive T helper (Th) 1 cells, which secrete inflammatory mediators such as interferon gamma. Type 3 immunity protects from extracellular bacteria and fungi using Type 3 innate lymphoid cells, Th17 cells and the cytokines interleukin (IL)-17 and IL-22. A type 2 immune response, in contrast, is characterized by tissue eosinophilia and elevated type 2 cytokines such as IL-4, IL-5, and IL-13. Typically, type 2 responses are associated with protection from venoms, parasites, environmental irritants, as well as fungi; however, it is also associated with allergies, CRS, and asthma.[7] Because more has been learned about airway inflammatory pathologic conditions, the importance of categorizing conditions such as CRS and asthma based on their inflammatory profile has become apparent.

Immune responses within the unified airway consist of both innate and adaptive pathways. Exposure to microbes, including fungi, initially induces an innate immune response, followed by the development of an adaptive immune response. The epithelium forms the first line of the innate defense and provides a physical barrier against the invasion of pathogens. The epithelium is connected via tight junctions that prevent invasion. It also produces mucus, which works together with cilia to physically remove pathogens. Further, epithelial cells express receptors that directly interact with microbes, resulting in the release of a class of cytokines and proinflammatory molecules called alarmins.[8] Alarmins include thymic stromal lymphopoietin (TSLP), IL-33, and IL-25.[9] Alarmins stimulate group 2 innate lymphoid cells (ILC2s) and contribute to both rapid type 2 cytokine (IL-4, IL-5, and IL-13) responses as well as tissue remodeling and fibrosis.[10] Granulocytes such as neutrophils and eosinophils contribute to innate immunity by both phagocytosing and degranulating in response to fungal antigens. Dendritic cells act as a bridge between innate and adaptive immunity by taking up local antigens and migrating to lymph nodes where they promote the differentiation of naïve T cells.

Adaptive immune responses rely on T cells and B cells, which develop antigen-specific surface receptors to combat pathogens. As with innate immunity, the epithelium plays a large role with the release of the alarmins TSLP, IL-25, and IL-33 after exposure to antigens.[11] These cytokines stimulate ILC2s to promote the differentiation of Th2-type CD4+ T cells, which in turn produce the cytokines IL-4, IL-5, and IL-13. These cytokines are responsible for a myriad of processes including class switching to immunoglobulin (Ig) E, production of IgG4, and goblet cell metaplasia of the airway epithelium. These changes result in enhanced mucus secretion (via IL-4 and IL-13), activation of eosinophils (via IL-5), and upregulation of vascular cell adhesion molecule 1[12] resulting in the activation of eosinophils, mast cells, and basophils.

Although type 2 inflammatory responses have been established as contributors to airway inflammation, recently the role of Th17 cells and the type 3 immune response to fungal elements has been elucidated. These cells are largely found in the intestinal and epidermal tissues and their dysregulation is seen in many local inflammatory disorders such as chronic obstructive pulmonary disease, inflammatory bowel disease, and cancer.[13] The Th17 response is particularly important in the response to *Candida albicans* because *C albicans*-specific Th17 cells are found in virtually all healthy patients.[13] Thus, it is likely that a combination of reduced Th17/type 3 responses with an increased type 2 response may characterize the inflammatory profile of patients with diseases such as AFRS. Additionally, Th17 signaling pathways have been shown to be a key contributor to the mechanism of severe asthma with elevated Th17-related cytokines consistently found in patients with severe asthma.[14]

FUNGAL COMPONENTS CAPABLE OF ACTIVATING TYPE 2 IMMUNE RESPONSE

CRSwNP, AFRS, allergic asthma, and other respiratory diseases with fungal type 2 immune reactions are due to both the infectious process as well as hypersensitivity responses to fungal elements. In recent years, the enzymatic processes by which these reactions take place have been identified. Fungal proteinases can induce both an allergic response to fungi as well as activate the innate immune system meant to limit fungal growth and local invasion.[15] These pathways are driven by fibrinogen cleavage products, cleaved from fibrinogen by fungal-specific proteinases.[16] These products then interact with toll-like receptor 4 and Mac-1 to initiate the signaling cascade that results in the characteristic airway hypersensitivity, neutrophilia, and eosinophilia seen in allergic airway disease.[15] Different fungal proteases have been shown to act through various pathways to elicit a fungal-mediated type 2 immune response. The release of IL-33, an alarmin involved in ILC2 stimulation has been linked to multiple fungal species. Significant, early IL-33 release and resulting pulmonary inflammation/asthma was shown to be caused by *Alternaria alternata*-derived serine proteases in a murine model.[17] Additionally, Luong and colleagues, demonstrated a protease activated receptor 2 (PAR2)-dependent IL-33 induction by *Aspergillus fumigatus* proteases in an in vitro human study using sinonasal epithelial cells.[18]

Although proteases have been shown to drive type 2-mediated immune responses in species such as *Alternaria* and *Aspergillus niger*, there are other fungal peptides that elicit Th2 and Th17 responses. One such peptide, a toxin known as candidalysin, is secreted by *C albicans* and drives the expression of airway mycosis symptoms but also functions to eradicate fungus and prevent invasion and dissemination of further fungal organisms.[13] It acts through a cascade of interactions that culminates in the release of the protein Dickkopf-1 (Dkk-1) by binding the Von Willebrand factor receptor glycoprotein 1bα (GP1bα) found on platelets. Dkk-1 is a Wnt pathway antagonist that stimulates Th2 and Th17 cell responses during airway mycosis. It seems as if the precursors to platelets, megakaryocytes, also express GP1bα receptors. These megakaryocytes, however, do not release Dkk-1 when exposed to candidalysin but assist in sequestering Dkk-1 into platelets, priming the release of Dkk-1 from platelets when exposed to candidalysin. Because *C albicans* has been isolated in up to two-thirds of asthma sputum samples and is capable of triggering airway hyperresponsiveness (AHR),[13] this protein may be an area of future study.

Similar to other pathogens, the structural polysaccharides of fungal cell walls seem to be a driver of immunologic response. Chitin is the second most common polysaccharide in nature and is present in the cell walls or exoskeletons of fungi, crustaceans, parasites, and insects.[19,20] In human airway epithelial cells, the surface receptor lysin motif domain 3 (LYSMD3) contains a LysM domain that binds the chitin of fungal cell walls.[19] This is of particular importance because the 3 alarmins associated with ILC2 activation, TSLP, IL-25, and IL-33 have been induced by chitin in murine models.[21] This again represents a promising target for future therapies. In fact, knock out of LYSMD3 reduced *Alternaria*-induced IL-33 release by human bronchial epithelial cells in vitro.[19]

Although new pathways for fungal-induced inflammation continue to become known, **Fig. 1** highlights some of the signaling pathways contributing to the type 2 immune response characteristic of these fungal-mediated chronic inflammatory airway diseases.

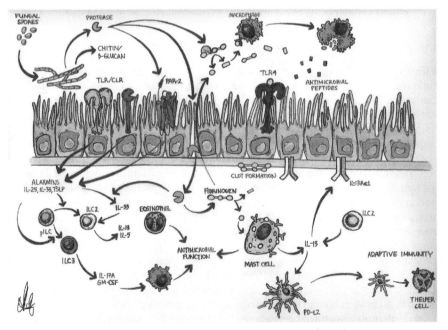

Fig. 1. Summary of innate and adaptive immune responses to fungal pathogens. (Image Courtesy: Dr. Shaina Gong, MD.)

PULMONARY MANIFESTATIONS OF FUNGAL-MEDIATED INFLAMMATION

The most common manifestation of human fungal illness, with the possible exception of cutaneous disease, is infectious complications involving the respiratory system. Highly lethal, invasive fungal infections of the lower airway, for example, invasive pulmonary aspergillosis, receive disproportionate attention relative to their rarity. Medically more significant are noninvasive inflammatory diseases of the lower airways that affect a substantial fraction of the population, and which are acquired by inhalation of ubiquitous fungal spores. Collectively referred to as airway mycosis-related disorders, these usually chronic fungal-related pulmonary syndromes comprise some of the most common disorders of humanity.[22,23] The 3 main airway mycosis-related pulmonary syndromes include allergic bronchopulmonary mycosis (ABPM; ABPA if the cause is an *Aspergillus* species), severe asthma with fungal sensitization (SAFS), and fungal asthma without fungal sensitization (FAWFS).

Regardless of the classification, most patients with asthma have AHR, the propensity to develop recurrent bouts of dyspnea that may be spontaneous or provoked by exposure to diverse allergens and respiratory irritants. AHR-related dyspnea is largely due to bronchial constriction, a complex physiologic response of the airway that is conditioned by the cytokines, IL-4, IL-13, and IL-17,[24,25] but directly mediated by cholinergic parasympathetic efferent nerves, especially from the vagus nerve,[26] and airway fibrinogen and thrombin.[27] Additional factors that enhance airway obstruction and dyspnea in asthma include goblet cell metaplasia and exaggerated mucus secretion, both of which are also conditioned by IL-4 and IL-13,[28] and plastic bronchitis, the production of fibrin clots in the airway.[29] Inflammatory exudate consisting largely of eosinophils and neutrophils that is often present in the asthmatic airway lumen may also impair air movement and gas exchange, thereby contributing to dyspnea.

Clinically, it is not possible to distinguish ABPM, SAFS, and FAWFS; rather these fungal syndromes are distinguished by immunologic and radiographic features. For example, ABPM, arguably the most severe of these conditions, is further characterized by radiographic abnormalities such as fleeting alveolar infiltrates and bronchiectasis; immunologic abnormalities that include very high total and fungus-specific IgE as well as fungus-specific IgG (formerly termed precipitins); and peripheral blood eosinophilia.[30] SAFS shares these features except for fungus-specific IgG and the radiographic abnormalities.[31] Total and fungal-specific IgE levels are typically lower in SAFS[32] compared with ABPM. Subjects with FAWFS most closely resemble those with SAFS but by definition fail to exhibit fungal sensitization.[22] Unfortunately, sputum fungal cultures are rarely performed due to their low yields when performed according to standard laboratory culture protocols.[33] However, multiple groups have documented improved fungal yields from sputum using updated methods.[33,34] For example, our method yields fungal growth from up to 87% of asthma sputum samples after a single culture.[23] This exceptionally high yield led to the discovery of the FAWFS subgroup of fungal asthma.

Because asthma and sputum fungal culture positivity are the only features that unite ABPM, SAFS and FAWFS, a fascinating and incompletely resolved question is why these disorders can be distinguished at all. The generally greater immune response against fungi and lung damage as documented radiographically suggest that ABPM reflects a more severe syndrome as compared with SAFS and FAWFS but the reason why fungal asthma is more severe in some patients remains unknown. Factors such as the virulence of the infecting fungi, medication use history, especially immunosuppressive corticosteroids, and subtle host immune defects could all be contributory elements. Equally unknown is why some patients with asthma manifest fungal sensitization, whereas patients with FAWFS do not. However, the vast majority of the many hundreds of fungi that are pathogenic for humans and potentially capable of causing airway mycosis are not represented in standard fungal sensitization assays, suggesting that incomplete testing for fungal culprits is a major factor.

SINONASAL MANIFESTATION OF FUNGI-MEDIATED INFLAMMATION

The sinonasal manifestations of fungal-mediated chronic inflammation are broad, ranging from colonization, fungal allergies, mycetomas (fungal balls), AFRS to CRSwNP. The particular manifestation experienced by each patient is largely dictated by the patient's local and systemic immune status.

As seen in the pulmonary system, acute invasive fungal rhinosinusitis can occur and is typically found in those with a compromised immune system. This diagnosis carries a high mortality (20%–80%) but is exceedingly rare (estimated 340 cases in 2018).[35] In patients with an intact immune system, fungal colonization can occur. Typically occurring after sinus surgery, the postoperative crusting can provide an environment favorable for replication of fungal species. This typically resolves after the removal of these crusts at routine postoperative visits.[36]

AR to fungal triggers is a result of clinically relevant amounts of fungal exposure limited to the nasal cavity[37] in sensitized individuals. This triggers a local type 2 response and IgE-mediated reactions that culminate in the degranulation of mast cells and basophils.[37] AR may be treated with exposure avoidance and pharmacologically can be managed with nasal corticosteroids, antihistamines, and allergen immunotherapy.

Fungal balls, conversely, have no preexisting atopic response to the fungal exposure but generate a mild inflammatory reaction to trapped germinated fungi within affected paranasal sinuses. These most commonly occur in the maxillary sinus and are thought to be due to inadequate mucociliary clearance of fungal species deposited in the sinus via normal respiration.[38] These present as a dense accumulation of fungal elements within a single paranasal sinus and are treated surgically by opening of the natural sinus ostia and evacuation of fungal elements. These do not typically require further treatment with surgical cure rates reaching 100%.[38,39]

AFRS is a subtype of CRSwNP that is characterized by eosinophilic mucin within expanded sinus cavities and IgE-mediated type 1 hypersensitivity to fungal elements.[40] These patients typically have an intact immune system but are now thought to have a local antifungal deficiency. Recent studies have demonstrated a deficiency of antimicrobial peptides (AMPs) in patients with AFRS when compared with patients with CRSwNP. Histatins are a family of 5 peptides spliced from 2 histatin genes originally found in the oral cavity associated with wound healing as well as antibacterial and antifungal properties.[41] Histatins have been shown to limit colonization of fungal species (eg, *C albicans*) on epithelial surfaces[42,43] and patients with AFRS have demonstrated a significant downregulation of expression of both histatin genes relative to other non-AFRS patients with nasal polyps.[44] Thus, because patients with AFRS have a locally decreased level of AMPs such as histatins, their sinuses present an environment more favorable for fungal proliferation.

The role of fungi in CRSwNP not meeting diagnostic criteria for AFRS remains unclear. Using updated methods to process nasal and sinus mucus, up to 97.5% of patients with CRS without AFRS have been shown to demonstrate growth on fungal culture and presence of fungal elements.[45,46] However, unlike AFRS, type 2 memory to the fungi was found in approximately 65% versus 100% in patients with AFRS.[22] Unlike AFRS, there is an upregulated expression of local AMPs, including histatins, in CRSwNP, which may limit the exposure and germination of fungal spores within the sinus cavity, and thereby limit contributory effects of fungi to the immune response. Both patients with CRSwNP and patients with AFRS can be managed with a combination of surgical and medical therapies, which have been another area of recent innovation. **Table 1** lists these common pulmonary and sinonasal fugal-associated diseases along with their clinical features and diagnostic characteristics.

TREATMENT IMPLICATIONS

Currently, there is no therapy that will reverse the underlying inflammatory processes associated with the reactive conditions of the unified airway. Similar to other forms of asthma and CRS, treatment of fungi-mediated chronic respiratory diseases often includes saline irrigations for the sinonasal region, beta-2 agonist for the lower airway, and topical corticosteroids for both. However, recent advancements in our understanding of these conditions have influenced the treatment paradigm for both sinonasal and pulmonary manifestations of fungi-mediated inflammation.

For AFRS (the primary sinonasal presentation of airway mycosis), sinus surgery is indicated earlier than in the treatment of other CRSwNP. This facilitates both the removal of thick, fungi-laden eosinophilic mucin and debris and improves penetration of saline irrigations and topical medications.[47] In the past, long-term, high-dose oral corticosteroids were a hallmark of AFRS management. Recent studies have demonstrated dose and duration-dependent adverse outcomes related to such high-dose corticosteroid use, including hyperglycemia, infection, poor wound healing, avascular necrosis.[48,49] As such, for patients with CRSwNP and AFRS, the current standard of care consists of a combination of surgery with nasal saline irrigations as well as maintenance topical corticosteroid rinses. Limited courses of oral corticosteroids are used for exacerbations. It should be noted that investigations into the effects of medical treatment of asthma or CRS with traditional therapies and its influences on the course of concurrent airway disease have been inconclusive.[50–52] These studies, however, did not focus on fungal-specific causes of airway disease.

To expand on treatments for asthma, CRS, and AFRS, alternative therapies are the subject of active study. As with other inflammatory conditions, the use of biologics targeting various points in the inflammatory cascade has been a recent focus of investigation. Several biologics targeting type 2 inflammatory mediators are currently available for the treatment of asthma, CRS, and AFRS recalcitrant to first-line therapies. There are currently multiple biologics approved for the treatment of asthma. Omalizumab (anti-IgE),[53] mepolizumab, reslizumab (anti-IL-5), benralizumab (anti-IL-5 receptor),[54] dupilumab (anti-IL-4 and anti-IL-13—targeting the shared IL-4α receptor),[55] and tezepelumab (anti-TSLP)[56] have all shown benefit in the treatment of asthmatics. Currently, omalizumab, dupilumab, and mepolizumab are approved for the treatment of CRSwNP after phase III studies demonstrated efficacious outcomes over placebo.[57–59] Clinical data for these biologics in the setting of fungi-mediated chronic respiratory diseases are less robust but beginning to accumulate.

For ABPM and SAFS, published experience primarily consisting of case reports and case series is available for omalizumab, mepolizumab, benralizumab, and dupilumab, with most studies available for omalizumab. In general, these biologics seem to reduce rates of exacerbations and decreased steroid use but the improvement in patient-reported outcomes and lung function is mixed.[60]

Similarly, less clinical experience with biologics is available for AFRS because these patients were excluded from pivotal phase III studies for severe CRSwNP. In general, several case reports and case series with dupilumab, mepolizumab, and omalizumab in AFRS demonstrated improvement in both objective and subjective outcome

Table 1
Sinonasal and pulmonary manifestation of fungi-mediated inflammation

	Disease Entity	Clinical Features	Diagnostic Characteristics
Sinonasal	AR with fungal sensitivity	*Symptoms*: nasal congestion, clear rhinorrhea, sneezing, postnasal drip, and nasal pruritis *Nasal endoscopy*: pale nasal mucosa and clear mucus	Clinical diagnosis Can perform fungal-specific IgE or allergy skin testing if empiric therapy fails
	Fungal ball (mycetoma)	*Symptoms*: typically, asymptomatic; may present with facial pain or nasal drainage	*CT findings*: unilateral sinus opacification with/without calcifications
	AFRS	*Nasal endoscopy*: polyposis and eosinophilic mucin	*CT findings*: serpiginous areas of high attenuation Positive fungal stain Elevated fungal IgE
	CRSwNP	*Symptoms*: mucoid nasal drainage, facial pressure/pain, nasal obstruction, and hyposmia *Nasal endoscopy*: polyposis and mucosal inflammation	*CT findings*: sinus opacification/mucosal thickening
Pulmonary	SAFS	*Symptoms*: wheezing, cough, dyspnea, and pleuritic chest pain	Elevated total IgE, fungal-specific IgE, or allergy skin testing
	FAWFS	*Symptoms*: wheezing, cough, dyspnea, and pleuritic chest pain	Normal fungal-specific IgE and allergy skin testing
	ABPM	*Symptoms*: wheezing, cough, dyspnea, pleuritic chest pain, and sputum with brown mucus plugs	Elevated total IgE, fungal-specific IgE, or allergy skin testing. *Radiographic findings*: alveolar infiltrates and bronchiectasis

measures including endoscopic modified Lung-Kennedy scores, computed tomography (CT) findings, and Sino-nasal outcome test 22 (SNOT-22) scores.[61–64] Compared with other CRS subtypes, AFRS is associated with exaggerated serum IgE levels.[65] A recent single-blind, randomized control trial by Mostafa and colleagues demonstrated a significant improvement in SNOT-20 scores, total nasal symptom scores and IgE but no difference in the endoscopic staging scores 6 months after a single dose of omalizumab compared with those treated with intranasal corticosteroids alone.[66] Overall, prospective randomized clinical trials are lacking in fungi-mediated chronic respiratory diseases but current clinical data and experience suggest a positive effect on several objective and subjective clinical endpoints with currently available biologics. Several clinical trials with this patient population are currently ongoing.

Although select biologics show promise in the management of AFRS and severe asthma, they, similar to corticosteroids and most other therapies, do not address the fundamental underlying cause of disease for these patients, which is airway mycosis. Antifungals have been recommended against, in general, CRS based on clinical trials with nonselective inclusion criteria.[67] However, studies (primarily case reports and case series) focused on AFRS or airway-mycosis associated CRSwNP show more positive although mixed results. One such study found significant improvements in both endoscopic and radiographic findings 24 weeks after surgery in patients with AFRS treated with both preoperative and postoperative itraconazole compared with steroids alone.[68] A recent retrospective study evaluated objective mucosal thickening changes following 4 to 12 weeks of antifungal treatment as noted by CT scan in 40 patients with airway mycosis-associated CRSwNP. Reduction in mucosal thickening was demonstrated in 75% of patients.[69] However, Rojita and colleagues found that if given itraconazole for 6 months at half the recommended dose (100 mg twice daily), patients with AFRS showed no improvement in any parameters postoperatively.[70] These studies indicate that itraconazole and other antifungals may be effective in select CRSwNP and AFRS but dosing and duration need to be optimized and prospective trials are needed.

Antifungal trials in fungi-mediated severe asthma have more consistently demonstrated durable benefits, including long-term disease remission. Stevens, and colleagues showed that itraconazole taken for 16 weeks resulted in clinically significant reductions in corticosteroid dose (>50%), or serum IgE (25% reduction), or minimum 25% improvements in exercise tolerance, pulmonary function tests, or pulmonary infiltrates in 46% of study subjects as compared with 19% of control subjects ($P = .04$) with no relapses after an additional 16 weeks of follow-up.[71] Similar positive outcomes with itraconazole were reported by Denning and colleagues in subjects with SAFS, with positive responses found in approximately 60% of subjects.[72] Additionally, fluconazole has been prospectively shown to be highly effective in asthma subjects with concomitant trichophyton dermatitis[73] and retrospective studies indicate that terbinafine and voriconazole can be effective as well.[74]

Although most patients with asthma and CRS tolerate oral antifungals well, systemic side effects can be clinically significant, sparking interest in topical AMPs as a treatment modality. These peptides have demonstrated antibiofilm properties that could prove beneficial to those with sinus disease.[75,76] In a murine model for rhinosinusitis, topical synthetic AMPs were shown to reduce nasal bacterial load and reduce inflammatory marker IL-6 (associated with nasal polyp formation).[76] The importance of biofilm formation in CRS and AFRS suggest AMPs may represents a low-risk treatment of patients with CRS and that there may be a role for antifungals in the management of AFRS.

FUTURE DIRECTIONS

Although much has been elucidated in recent years regarding the role of fungus in reactive airway disease in the unified airway, many questions remain. Understanding the underlying mechanisms that explain the local (antifungal deficiencies in AFRS) and systemic immune abnormalities (hyperactive type 2 responses) that contribute to various reactive airway disease in both the upper and lower airways may present new targets for therapies. As of now, there are multiple potential targets worthy of investigation. As previously mentioned, the role of AMPs and their use as a treatment modality is largely unexplored and holds promise in the treatment of AFRS. Additionally, the identification of pathogenic molecules (protease, candidalysin, and chitin) and their immunogenic pathways (PAR2, GP1bα, and LYSMD3) present new avenues for potential therapeutics.

SUMMARY

The unified airway refers to the combined upper and lower airways and their shared pathophysiologic relationship, specifically related to inflammatory airway diseases of asthma, CRS, and AFRS. The pathophysiology of these diseases is defined by type 2 immunologic reactions, which have been better characterized in recent years. Additionally, the pathogenic components of fungi have been better identified with proteases, candidalysin, and chitin all representing unique pathways and potential targets for future therapies. Current therapies consist of a combination of steroids, saline irrigations, surgery, biologics, and beta agonists (for asthma); however, novel understandings of the molecular signaling of fungi contributory to the inflammatory changes in the unified airway provide opportunities for novel and targeted therapeutics.

CONFLICT OF INTEREST

A.U. Luong serves as a consultant for Lyra Therapeutics (Watertown, MA, USA), Medtronic (Dublin, IE), NeuroENT (Galway, IE), Sanofi (Paris, France), and Stryker (Kalamazoo, MI, USA). A.U. Luong serves on the scientific advisory board for ENTvantage Dx (Austin, TX, USA), Maxwell Biosciences (Austin, TX), and SoundHealth (San Francisco, CA, USA). D.B. Corry serves as a consultant for Maxwell Biosciences (Austin, TX) and owns intellectual property through Fannin Innovation Studio and Baylor College of Medicine.

REFERENCES

1. Licari A, Castagnoli R, Denicolo CF, et al. The Nose and the Lung: United Airway Disease? Front Pediatr 2017;5:44.
2. Khan AH, Gouia I, Kamat S, et al. Prevalence and Severity Distribution of Type 2 Inflammation-Related Comorbidities Among Patients with Asthma, Chronic Rhinosinusitis with Nasal Polyps, and Atopic Dermatitis. Lung 2023;201(1):57–63.
3. Promsopa C, Kansara S, Citardi MJ, et al. Prevalence of confirmed asthma varies in chronic rhinosinusitis subtypes. Int Forum Allergy Rhinol 2016;6(4):373–7.
4. Woodcock A. Moulds and asthma: time for indoor climate change? Thorax 2007; 62(9):745–6.
5. AlQahtani A, Alim B, Almudhaibery F, et al. The Impact of Climatic, Socioeconomic, and Geographic Factors on the Prevalence of Allergic Fungal Rhinosinusitis: A Worldwide Ecological Study. Am J Rhinol Allergy 2022. https://doi.org/10. 1177/19458924211069226. 19458924211069226.
6. Ferguson BJ, Barnes L, Bernstein JM, et al. Geographic variation in allergic fungal rhinosinusitis. Otolaryngol Clin North Am 2000;33(2):441–9.
7. Annunziato F, Romagnani C, Romagnani S. The 3 major types of innate and adaptive cell-mediated effector immunity. J Allergy Clin Immunol 2015;135(3):626–35.
8. Schleimer RP, Kato A, Kern R, et al. Epithelium: at the interface of innate and adaptive immune responses. J Allergy Clin Immunol 2007;120(6):1279–84.
9. Roan F, Obata-Ninomiya K, Ziegler SF. Epithelial cell-derived cytokines: more than just signaling the alarm. J Clin Invest 2019;129(4):1441–51.
10. Kindermann M, Knipfer L, Atreya I, et al. ILC2s in infectious diseases and organ-specific fibrosis. Semin Immunopathol 2018;40(4):379–92.
11. Akdis M, Aab A, Altunbulakli C, et al. Interleukins (from IL-1 to IL-38), interferons, transforming growth factor beta, and TNF-alpha: Receptors, functions, and roles in diseases. J Allergy Clin Immunol 2016;138(4):984–1010.
12. Lavigne P, Lee SE. Immunomodulators in chronic rhinosinusitis. World J Otorhinolaryngol Head Neck Surg 2018;4(3):186–92.
13. Wu Y, Zeng Z, Guo Y, et al. Candida albicans elicits protective allergic responses via platelet mediated T helper 2 and T helper 17 cell polarization. Immunity 2021; 54(11):2595–2610 e7.

14. Ramakrishnan RK, Al Heialy S, Hamid Q. Role of IL-17 in asthma pathogenesis and its implications for the clinic. Expert Rev Respir Med 2019;13(11):1057–68.
15. Haruna S, Takeda K, El-Hussien MA, et al. Local production of broadly cross-reactive IgE against multiple fungal cell wall polysaccharides in patients with allergic fungal rhinosinusitis. Allergy 2022;77(10):3147–51.
16. Millien VO, Lu W, Shaw J, et al. Cleavage of fibrinogen by proteinases elicits allergic responses through Toll-like receptor 4. Science 2013;341(6147):792–6.
17. Snelgrove RJ, Gregory LG, Peiro T, et al. Alternaria-derived serine protease activity drives IL-33-mediated asthma exacerbations. J Allergy Clin Immunol 2014;134(3):583–592 e6.
18. Dietz CJ, Sun H, Yao WC, et al. Aspergillus fumigatus induction of IL-33 expression in chronic rhinosinusitis is PAR2-dependent. Laryngoscope 2019;129(10): 2230–5.
19. He X, Howard BA, Liu Y, et al. LYSMD3: A mammalian pattern recognition receptor for chitin. Cell Rep 2021;36(3):109392.
20. Lee CG. Chitin, chitinases and chitinase-like proteins in allergic inflammation and tissue remodeling. Yonsei Med J 2009;50(1):22–30.
21. Van Dyken SJ, Mohapatra A, Nussbaum JC, et al. Chitin activates parallel immune modules that direct distinct inflammatory responses via innate lymphoid type 2 and gammadelta T cells. Immunity 2014;40(3):414–24.
22. Porter PC, Lim DJ, Maskatia ZK, et al. Airway surface mycosis in chronic TH2-associated airway disease. J Allergy Clin Immunol 2014;134(2):325–31.
23. Li E, Knight JM, Wu Y, et al. Airway mycosis in allergic airway disease. Adv Immunol 2019;142:85–140.
24. Grünig G, Warnock M, Wakil AE, et al. Requirement for IL-13 independently of IL-4 in experimental asthma. Science 1998;282(5397):2261–3.
25. Kudo M, Melton AC, Chen C, et al. IL-17A produced by $\alpha\beta$ T cells drives airway hyper-responsiveness in mice and enhances mouse and human airway smooth muscle contraction. Nat Med 2012;18(4):547–54.
26. Hahn HL. Role of the parasympathetic nervous system and of cholinergic mechanisms in bronchial hyperreactivity. Bull Eur Physiopathol Respir 1986;22(Suppl 7):112–42.
27. Wagers SS, Norton RJ, Rinaldi LM, et al. Extravascular fibrin, plasminogen activator, plasminogen activator inhibitors, and airway hyperresponsiveness. J Clin Invest 2004;114(1):104–11.
28. Li E, Landers CT, Tung HY, et al. Fungi in Mucoobstructive Airway Diseases. Ann Am Thorac Soc 2018;15(Suppl 3):S198–204.
29. Panchabhai TS, Mukhopadhyay S, Sehgal S, et al. Plugs of the Air Passages: A Clinicopathologic Review. Chest 2016;150(5):1141–57.
30. Shah A, Panjabi C. Allergic Bronchopulmonary Aspergillosis: A Perplexing Clinical Entity. Allergy Asthma Immunol Res 2016;8(4):282–97.
31. Agarwal R. Severe asthma with fungal sensitization. Curr Allergy Asthma Rep 2011;11(5):403–13.
32. Hogan C, Denning DW. Allergic bronchopulmonary aspergillosis and related allergic syndromes. Semin Respir Crit Care Med 2011;32(6):682–92.
33. Mak G, Porter PC, Bandi V, et al. Tracheobronchial mycosis in a retrospective case-series study of five status asthmaticus patients. Clin Immunol 2013; 146(2):77–83.
34. Pashley CH, Fairs A, Morley JP, et al. Routine processing procedures for isolating filamentous fungi from respiratory sputum samples may underestimate fungal prevalence. Med Mycol 2012;50(4):433–8.

35. Shintani-Smith S, Luong AU, Ramakrishnan VR, et al. Acute invasive fungal sinusitis: Epidemiology and outcomes in the United States. Int Forum Allergy Rhinol. Feb 2022;12(2):233–6.

36. Soler ZM, Schlosser RJ. The role of fungi in diseases of the nose and sinuses. Am J Rhinol Allergy 2012;26(5):351–8.

37. Twaroch TE, Curin M, Valenta R, et al. Mold allergens in respiratory allergy: from structure to therapy. Allergy Asthma Immunol Res 2015;7(3):205–20.

38. Nicolai P, Lombardi D, Tomenzoli D, et al. Fungus ball of the paranasal sinuses: experience in 160 patients treated with endoscopic surgery. Laryngoscope 2009; 119(11):2275–9.

39. Lee KC. Clinical features of the paranasal sinus fungus ball. J Otolaryngol 2007; 36(5):270–3.

40. Cameron BH, Luong AU. New Developments in Allergic Fungal Rhinosinusitis Pathophysiology and Treatment. Am J Rhinol Allergy 2023;37(2):214–20.

41. Zolin GVS, Fonseca FHD, Zambom CR, et al. Histatin 5 Metallopeptides and Their Potential against Candida albicans Pathogenicity and Drug Resistance. Biomolecules 2021;11(8):1209.

42. Bacher P, Hohnstein T, Beerbaum E, et al. Human Anti-fungal Th17 Immunity and Pathology Rely on Cross-Reactivity against Candida albicans. Cell 2019;176(6): 1340–1355 e15.

43. Torres P, Castro M, Reyes M, et al. Histatins, wound healing, and cell migration. Oral Dis 2018;24(7):1150–60.

44. Tyler MA, Padro Dietz CJ, Russell CB, et al. Distinguishing Molecular Features of Allergic Fungal Rhinosinusitis. Otolaryngol Head Neck Surg 2018;159(1):185–93.

45. Guo C, Ghadersohi S, Kephart GM, et al. Improving the detection of fungi in eosinophilic mucin: seeing what we could not see before. Otolaryngol Head Neck Surg 2012;147(5):943–9.

46. JU Ponikau, Sherris DA, Kern EB, et al. The diagnosis and incidence of allergic fungal sinusitis. Mayo Clin Proc 1999;74(9):877–84.

47. Medikeri G, Javer A. Optimal Management of Allergic Fungal Rhinosinusitis. J Asthma Allergy 2020;13:323–32.

48. Poetker DM. Oral corticosteroids in the management of chronic rhinosinusitis with and without nasal polyps: Risks and benefits. Am J Rhinol Allergy 2015;29(5): 339–42.

49. Poetker DM, Smith TL. Medicolegal Implications of Common Rhinologic Medications. Otolaryngol Clin North Am 2015;48(5):817–26.

50. Ragab S, Parikh A, Darby YC, et al. An open audit of montelukast, a leukotriene receptor antagonist, in nasal polyposis associated with asthma. Clin Exp Allergy 2001;31(9):1385–91.

51. Schaper C, Noga O, Koch B, et al. Anti-inflammatory properties of montelukast, a leukotriene receptor antagonist in patients with asthma and nasal polyposis. J Investig Allergol Clin Immunol 2011;21(1):51–8.

52. American Lung Association-Asthma Clinical Research Centers' Writing C, Dixon AE, Castro M, et al. Efficacy of nasal mometasone for the treatment of chronic sinonasal disease in patients with inadequately controlled asthma. J Allergy Clin Immunol 2015;135(3):701–709 e5.

53. Hanania NA, Alpan O, Hamilos DL, et al. Omalizumab in severe allergic asthma inadequately controlled with standard therapy: a randomized trial. Ann Intern Med 2011;154(9):573–82.

54. Wang FP, Liu T, Lan Z, et al. Efficacy and Safety of Anti-Interleukin-5 Therapy in Patients with Asthma: A Systematic Review and Meta-Analysis. PLoS One 2016;11(11):e0166833.
55. Wenzel S, Ford L, Pearlman D, et al. Dupilumab in persistent asthma with elevated eosinophil levels. N Engl J Med 2013;368(26):2455–66.
56. Corren J, Parnes JR, Wang L, et al. Tezepelumab in Adults with Uncontrolled Asthma. N Engl J Med 2017;377(10):936–46.
57. Bachert C, Han JK, Desrosiers M, et al. Efficacy and safety of dupilumab in patients with severe chronic rhinosinusitis with nasal polyps (LIBERTY NP SINUS-24 and LIBERTY NP SINUS-52): results from two multicentre, randomised, double-blind, placebo-controlled, parallel-group phase 3 trials. Lancet 2019;394(10209): 1638–50.
58. Gevaert P, Omachi TA, Corren J, et al. Efficacy and safety of omalizumab in nasal polyposis: 2 randomized phase 3 trials. J Allergy Clin Immunol 2020;146(3): 595–605.
59. Han JK, Bachert C, Fokkens W, et al. Mepolizumab for chronic rhinosinusitis with nasal polyps (SYNAPSE): a randomised, double-blind, placebo-controlled, phase 3 trial. Lancet Respir Med 2021;9(10):1141–53.
60. Moss RB. Severe Fungal Asthma: A Role for Biologics and Inhaled Antifungals. J Fungi (Basel) 2023;9(1):85.
61. Mujahed RA, Marglani OA, Maksood LS, et al. Successful Use of Dupilumab as a Salvage Therapy for Recalcitrant Allergic Fungal Rhinosinusitis: A Case Report. Cureus 2022;14(3):e23104.
62. Alotaibi NH, Aljasser LA, Arnaout RK, et al. A case report of allergic fungal rhinosinusitis managed with Dupilumab. Int J Surg Case Rep 2021;88:106479.
63. Bulkhi AA, Mirza AA, Aburiziza AJ, et al. Dupilumab: An emerging therapy in allergic fungal rhinosinusitis. World Allergy Organ J 2022;15(3):100638.
64. Karp J, Dhillon I, Panchmatia R, et al. Subcutaneous Mepolizumab Injection: An Adjunctive Treatment for Recalcitrant Allergic Fungal Rhinosinusitis Patients With Asthma. Am J Rhinol Allergy 2021;35(2):256–63.
65. Hutcheson PS, Schubert MS, Slavin RG. Distinctions between allergic fungal rhinosinusitis and chronic rhinosinusitis. Am J Rhinol Allergy. Nov-Dec 2010;24(6): 405–8.
66. Mostafa BE, Fadel M, Mohammed MA, et al. Omalizumab versus intranasal steroids in the post-operative management of patients with allergic fungal rhinosinusitis. Eur Arch Oto-Rhino-Laryngol 2020;277(1):121–8.
67. Head K, Sharp S, Chong LY, et al. Topical and systemic antifungal therapy for chronic rhinosinusitis. Cochrane Database Syst Rev 2018;9(9):CD012453.
68. Verma RK, Patro SK, Francis AA, et al. Role of preoperative versus postoperative itraconazole in allergic fungal rhinosinusitis. Med Mycol 2017;55(6):614–23.
69. Li E, Scheurer M, Kheradmand F, et al. Computer-Assisted Analysis of Oral Antifungal Therapy in Chronic Rhinosinusitis with Airway Mycosis: a Retrospective Cohort Analysis. Antimicrob Agents Chemother 2021;65(11):e0169721.
70. Rojita M, Samal S, Pradhan P, et al. Comparison of Steroid and Itraconazole for Prevention of Recurrence in Allergic Fungal Rhinosinusitis: A Randomized Controlled Trial. J Clin Diagn Res 2017;11(4):MC01–3.
71. Stevens DA, Schwartz HJ, Lee JY, et al. A randomized trial of itraconazole in allergic bronchopulmonary aspergillosis. N Engl J Med 2000;342:756–62.
72. Denning DW, O'Driscoll BR, Powell G, et al. Randomized controlled trial of oral antifungal treatment for severe asthma with fungal sensitization: The Fungal Asthma Sensitization Trial (FAST) study. Am J Respir Crit Care Med 2009;

179(1):11–8 [published correction appears in Am J Respir Crit Care Med. 2009;179(4):330-1].

73. Ward GW Jr, Woodfolk JA, Hayden ML, et al. Treatment of late-onset asthma with fluconazole. J Allergy Clin Immunol 1999;104(3 Pt 1):541–6.

74. Li E, Tsai CL, Maskatia ZK, et al. Benefits of antifungal therapy in asthma patients with airway mycosis: A retrospective cohort analysis. Immun Inflamm Dis 2018; 6(2):264–75.

75. Haney EF, Hancock RE. Peptide design for antimicrobial and immunomodulatory applications. Biopolymers 2013;100(6):572–83.

76. Alford MA, Choi KG, Trimble MJ, et al. Murine Model of Sinusitis Infection for Screening Antimicrobial and Immunomodulatory Therapies. Front Cell Infect Microbiol 2021;11:621081.

Air Quality, Allergic Rhinitis, and Asthma

Abdulrahman Alenezi, MD, FRCSC[a], Hannan Qureshi, MD[a],
Omar G. Ahmed, MD[b,c], Murugappan Ramanathan Jr, MD[a,*]

KEYWORDS

- Air quality • Air pollution • Allergic rhinitis • Asthma • Inflammation • Exacerbation
- Airway inflammation • TRAP

KEY POINTS

- Air pollution is a global problem with far reaching medical and health related concerns that affect individuals across all ages.
- Pathogenesis and exacerbation of upper and lower airway disease involves exposure to airborne pollutants.
- Early exposure of air pollution in the prenatal and early childhood period can be associated with long term development of allergic rhinitis and asthma.
- Chronic exposure to air pollution is associated with risk of increased exacerbations and emergency hospital visits in the pediatric population.

INTRODUCTION

The World Health Organization now recognizes air pollution as the largest environmental threat to human health in their most recent update on Global Air Quality Guidelines.[1] Air pollution, as a whole, refers to the contamination of the atmosphere caused by the introduction of chemical, biological, or physical substances into either indoor or outdoor environments.[2] The Environmental Protection Agency has outlined 6 criteria of air pollutants, namely ozone (O_3), particulate matter (PM), carbon onoxide (CO), lead (Pb), sulfur dioxide (SO2), and nitrogen dioxide (NO_2) in order to establish a set air quality standard in the United States.[3] PM has been further categorized based on size with a measure of diameter of 10 μm or less (PM_{10}) or 2.5 μm or less ($PM_{2.5}$), in order to distinguish its various effects on health.

Epidemiologically, there has been a growing body of evidence that highlights the effects of air pollutants on health and its impact on disease burden. For example, a

[a] Department of Otolaryngology- Head and Neck Surgery, Johns Hopkins School of Medicine, Johns Hopkins Outpatient Center, 6th Floor, 601 North Caroline Street, Baltimore, MD 21287-0910, USA; [b] Academic Institute, Houston, TX 77030, USA; [c] Research Institute, Otolaryngology-Head and Neck Surgery, Houston Methodist Hospital, Houston, TX 77030, USA
* Corresponding author.
E-mail address: mramana3@jhmi.edu

Otolaryngol Clin N Am 57 (2024) 293–307
https://doi.org/10.1016/j.otc.2023.10.005
0030-6665/24/© 2023 Elsevier Inc. All rights reserved.

recent meta-analysis by Orellano and colleagues revealed findings indicating a positive association between brief exposure to PM_{10}, $PM_{2.5}$, NO2, and O3 and increased all-cause mortality rates, as well as a correlation between PM_{10} and $PM_{2.5}$ exposure and higher incidences of cardiovascular, respiratory, and cerebrovascular deaths.[4]

This review aims to provide a comprehensive overview of the global impact of air pollution and its link to the pathogenesis and exacerbation of inflammatory sinonasal and airway disorders, particularly allergic rhinitis and asthma.

BACKGROUND AND PATHOGENESIS

The pathogenesis of sinonasal and chronic airway inflammatory disorders is complex, and multiple factors including the environment and air pollutants have been identified to play a significant role in either initiating or exacerbating these diseases. Pollutants can be divided into gaseous matter or PM based on particle size. Gaseous pollutants include inorganic substances such as NOSO, CO, O3, and carbon dioxide[5] On the other hand, PM are pollutants which are thought to have a greater impact on human health and are commonly used to measure air quality.[6] PM is categorized by size, where larger PM_{10} generally accumulate in the upper airway and can lead to the disruption of the nasal mucosa, as it is one of the first respiratory epithelial barriers.[7] In addition, smaller or finer PM, such as $PM_{2.5}$ or $PM_{0.1}$, are more likely to be deposited in lower airway such as the alveoli and terminal bronchioles, and can potentially cross the cell membrane if particulates are sized less than 0.1 μm.[8]

Air pollutants can exert their effects directly via oxidative stress by production of reactive oxygen species, diffusion from airway surfaces, or indirectly via induction of inflammation. Components of PM such as diesel emission particles (DEP), ultrafine particles, and $PM_{2.5}$, can act as allergen-like adjuvants. Such particles have redox-active metals, which can induce inflammation and oxidative stress shifting immune function from a T-helper cell type 1 (Th1) to a Th2 response, and in turn driving lymphocyte proliferation and IgE production.[9]

Traffic-related air pollution (TRAP), which includes pollutants such as nitrogen oxide and DEP, has also been strongly associated with asthma and lower airway disease.[10] In contrast to lower airway disease, the link between TRAP and allergic rhinitis has not been as well established.[11] That being said, there has been a growing body of evidence and interest in studying the relationship of development of allergic rhinitis and exposure to pollutants including TRAP. In a very recent systematic review published by Liu and colleagues, TRAP exposure in the prenatal period and first year of life was positively associated with development of allergic rhinitis in children.[12] Outdoor air pollution has also been studied across various pediatric and adult populations. A recent systematic review of the Latin American population found individuals exposed to pollutants had a 43% increased risk of developing allergic rhinitis.[13]

Other studies have looked at the effect of pollution in the development of both asthma and chronic obstructive pulmonary disease (COPD). For example, Lindgren and colleagues looked at annual mean level of nitrogen dioxide levels in Sweden and found adults that lived within 100m of a road with a traffic intensity (defined as >10 cars/min) had a 1.4 (95% CI, 1.04–1.89) and 1.64 (95% CI, 1.11–2.40) odds ratio of developing asthma and COPD, respectively.[10] In addition, a multicenter study based on 5 European birth cohorts from the European Study of Cohorts for Air Pollution Effects has shown poor lung outcomes in school-aged children with exposure to air pollutants such as PM and nitrogen oxides.[14] This has been further supported by other large observational epidemiologic studies, including a meta-analysis which showed a positive correlation between traffic pollution and childhood asthma.[15] There is also growing evidence of pollution exposure and the development of allergic rhinitis. A study based on children illustrated a positive correlation between the frequency of the episodes of allergic rhinitis and higher vehicular traffic and pollutant concentration of PM_{10}, nitrogen dioxide, and ozone levels.[12,14]

One of the major constituents of TRAP is the DEP pollutant which may potentially exacerbate allergic rhinitis. This has been studied in vivo in a murine model using mice sensitized to ragweed pollen and subsequently challenged with ragweed pollen in presence and absence of DEP. The study revealed that there was increased sneezing frequency in presence of DEP, indicating a possible exacerbation of allergic rhinitis symptoms.[16] DEP was also shown to increase disruption of the epithelial barrier in vitro due changes of the tight junction integrity. Kim and colleagues demonstrated increased expression of inflammatory cytokines interleukin-6 (IL-6) and interleukin-8 (IL-8) in DEP-stimulated nasal fibroblasts.[17] They further validated their findings in an ex vivo organ culture of the inferior turbinate. Due to the increase in pro-inflammatory cytokine expression, the study findings suggest possible effects of air pollution on induction or exacerbation of allergic rhinitis.[18]

Additionally, indoor pollution is also an important factor to be considered in the pathogenesis and association of air quality and sinonasal disorders and airway disease. It is composed of several components including the outdoor pollutants previously mentioned, indoor allergens, and byproducts of indoor activities such as smoking, heating, and cooking.[19] Of the indoor/outdoor pollutants, tobacco smoke has been established as toxic and detrimental to human health. Tobacco smoke includes at least 4500 toxic compounds that include PM, heavy metals, oxidative gases, and at least 50 carcinogens.[20] The mechanism by which smoking disrupts the sinonasal functions is multifactorial and includes disruption in key aspects of normal sinonasal activity such as mucociliary clearance, epithelial barrier, and vitamin d conversion. It also has the effect of increasing the oxidative stress and increasing inflammatory mediators.[21] Cigarette smoking has been shown to impair the ability of human sinonasal epithelial cells to convert of vitamin D3 to its active form, hence resulting in increased sinonasal epithelial release of pro-inflammatory cytokines.[21]

In vitro studies have also illustrated various detrimental effects of smoking on sinonasal epithelium. Lee and colleagues demonstrated cigarette smoke exposure impaired sinonasal epithelial growth and induced apoptosis of normal epithelial cells.[22] Furthermore, Cohen and colleagues illustrated cigarette smoke condensate reduced both ciliary beat frequency and transepithelial chloride transport, 2 of the major components of mucociliary clearance, in both human and murine derived cultures.[23] Disruption of the upper and lower airway epithelium and mucociliary clearance lead to exacerbations of sinonasal disease and chronic airway conditions such as asthma and COPD. These effects are a result of both active and passive smoke which is relevant to the adult and pediatric population. Moreover, secondhand smoke exposure during pregnancy and infancy has been associated with asthma onset, poor asthma control, and more pronounced exacerbations of episodes during childhood.[24] Although an abundance of evidence is present to describe the role of smoke in the pathogenesis of asthma and chronic sinonasal disorders, evidence is still lacking in establishing a significant association with allergic rhinitis. As per the most recent iteration of the International Consensus Statement on Allergy and Rhinology on Allergic Rhinitis, results from large prospective studies and systematic reviews have not shown a correlation between active and passive smoking and allergic rhinitis.[25]

Allergic Rhinitis

There is increasing evidence of the role of air pollution in both the development and exacerbation of rhinitis. There are several mechanisms believed to play a role of air pollution in the development of rhinitis. In vivo human studies have demonstrated the effect of pollutants in enhancing nasal cytokine expression and potentiation of allergen specific IgE production[26,27] Other in vivo studies, such as the one published by Ramanthan and colleagues, demonstrated the effect of chronic airborne $PM_{2.5}$ exposure on sinonasal epithelium with resultant disruption and increased accumulation of inflammatory cells and pro-inflammatory cytokines.[28] These mechanisms disrupt the epithelial barrier layer that protects the underlying sinonasal mucosa from the external environmental irritants which in turn contributes to the development of Rhinitis.[28]

Earlier studies in the literature found no significant association with the incidence of allergic rhinitis and the exposure of air pollution.[29] Gerhing and colleagues conducted a large population-based birth cohort study involving 14,126 participants to investigate the impact of air pollution exposure on the development of asthma and rhinoconjunctivitis, which tracked patients up to the age of 14 to 16 years and revealed a positive association between air pollution exposure, specifically nitric oxide levels and $PM_{2.5}$, and the occurrence of asthma.[30] However, no significant correlation was observed between air pollution exposure and the incidence of rhinoconjunctivitis.

However, more recent studies have produced evidence demonstrating effect of air pollution and sinonasal inflammation and rhinitis. As an example, using novel techniques that involve incorporating residential zip codes into a deep learning neural network model, Franks and colleagues were able to demonstrate the consistently higher levels of fine particulate matter ($PM_{2.5}$) in patients with non-allergic rhinitis in the 5 years preceding patients' diagnosis. The study presented findings that suggest an increased odd of developing non-allergic rhinitis that was associated with a 5 µg/m^3 increase in $PM_{2.5}$ concentration[31]

There is also growing evidence for an association between air pollution and specifically allergic rhinitis. In a recent systematic review and meta-analysis, Li and colleagues have evaluated 35 studies across 12 countries in Europe and Asia, reporting a positive association between air pollution and the prevalence of allergic rhinitis.[32] The review suggested that geographic locations and economic levels are possible modifiers to the association, where a stronger association was found in developing countries compared to developed ones.[32] Additionally, a meta-analysis by Zou and colleagues, demonstrated higher prevalence of allergic rhinitis with higher levels of air pollutants (NO_2, $PM2._5$, SO_2).[33] The effect of PM was further supported by findings reported by several studies, including one published by Teng and colleagues and a systematic review published by Lin and colleagues[34,35]

Given early development in childhood asthma and allergic rhinitis can have long-standing effects into adulthood; there has been a great focus on allergic rhinitis in the pediatric population and its association with air pollution. In a large Taiwanese cohort study of preschool children, the prevalence of allergic rhinitis was found to be about 10.9% with findings suggesting associations with CO and NO.[36] In another study based in Korea, near-road exposure and impact of air pollution on allergic disease in elementary school children demonstrated increased episodes of allergic rhinitis in relation to increase black carbon and SO_2 levels.[37] The impact of ambient air pollution has been investigated in a younger population as well. Liu and colleagues conducted a retrospective cohort study that revealed associations between allergic rhinitis, asthma, and gestational and early-life exposure to ambient NO2.[38]

In contrast, a positive association between other components of air pollution, such as tobacco smoke, and allergic rhinitis has not established. A large meta-analysis by Skaaby and colleagues found a lower risk of allergy sensitization and hay fever with current or previous smokers and an inverse dose-response relationship with smoking exposure and hay fever.[39] Another meta-analysis by Zhou and colleagues studied the effect of smoke exposure during pregnancy, suggesting maternal passive smoke exposure during pregnancy and not active smoking increases the risk of the offspring developing allergic rhinitis.[40] Further details on the effect of air pollution exposure are illustrated in **Table 1**.

Asthma

The effects of air pollution and its association with the development of respiratory diseases and conditions such as asthma have long been studied. Specifically the effects of pollution and its impact on asthma can be categorized by indoor versus outdoor sources such as tobacco smoking and TRAP.[24]

In a systematic review and meta-analysis by Khreis, specific exposure to TRAP and the development of asthma was evaluated with findings suggesting a positive correlation and statistical significance between $PM_{2.5}$, PM_{10}, NO_2 and development of asthma.[41] This is further supported by a recent meta-analysis that reviewed studies from 2000 to 2019 with results supporting the positive association between TRAP exposure and development of childhood asthma.[42]

Further studies looked into the that association with various asthma phenotypes, where in one study patients with asthma were categorized based on their age and duration of wheezing as one of 4 groups; (1) no wheezing, (2) transient wheezing (onset before the age of 3), (3) persistent wheezing (before the age of 3 and at the age of 6), and finally, (4) late onset wheezing (after the age of 6 only). In one study, findings suggested an association with TRAP exposure and the transient and persistent wheezing groups.[43]

The relationship of air pollution and asthma has been also studied at the earlier stages of life where the association of $PM_{2.5}$ and pregnancy and its effects on early life have been investigated. In a prospective birth cohort study that followed patients from early pregnancy to 3 to 4 years after birth over 3700 children were included, 10.52% of children were diagnosed with asthma, with positive association of prenatal and postnatal $PM_{2.5}$ exposure to the development of the disease. Further analysis revealed stronger association in the 6 to 24 gestational age and in the first 3 years of birth post-delivery.[44]

Similarly, studies were also conducted to evaluate the role of smoking, active and second-hand smoking, in the development of early childhood asthma. As previously described, smoking has been associated with poorer asthma outcomes, earlier onset and more severe exacerbations. In an analysis by Thacher and colleagues, 5 European birth cohorts with over 10,000 participants were studied for the effect of parental smoking on fetal life to adolescence on the development of asthma and rhinoconjunctivitis. In this study, a positive correlation was found between any parental smoking and the transient asthma phenotype development in children with findings of an association of persistent asthma with maternal smoking of over 10 cigarettes per day.[45]

As previously mentioned, there is a substantial body of evidence in the literature in regards to the effect of air pollution on the severity of asthma. This was demonstrated by multiple studies that investigated the rates of pediatric emergency department visits or hospital admissions and the potential effect of ambient air pollution. For an example, a time stratified case crossover study in Detroit, Michigan, revealed a positive effect between $PM_{2.5}$ concentrations and the rates of pediatric asthma related

Table 1
Allergic rhinitis and air pollution

Author/Year	Title	Number of Participants	Results/Conclusion
Li et al,[32] 2022	Association between exposure to air pollution and risk of allergic rhinitis: a systematic review and meta-analysis.	n = 453,470	• The OR per 10 μg/m3 increase of pollutants was 1.13 (1.04–1.22) for PM_{10} and 1.12 (1.05–1.20) for $PM_{2.5}$. • The OR per 10 μg/m3 increment of gaseous pollutants were 1.13 (1.07–1.20) for NO_2, 1.13 (1.04–1.22) for SO_2 and 1.07 (1.01–1.12) for O_3. • No significant association was observed between CO and AR. • Children or adolescents are more sensitive to air pollution than adults. • The effects of PM_{10} and SO_2 were significantly stronger in Europe than Asia. • The effects of air pollutants were more significant and higher in developing countries than in developed countries, except for PM_{10}. • A significant difference of subgroup test was found between developed and developing countries of NO_2.
Zou et al,[33] 2018	Exposure to air pollution and risk of prevalence of childhood allergic rhinitis: a meta-analysis.	n = 123,266	• Exposure to NO_2 OR Europe = 1.031, 95%CI [1.002,1.060], P = .033 • Exposure to NO_2 OR Asia = 1.236, 95%CI [1.099,1.390], P = .000 • Exposure to NO_2 OR overall = 1.138, 95%CI [1.052,1.231], P = .001) • Exposure to SO_2 OR Europe = 1.148, 95%CI [1.030,1.279], P = .012 • Exposure to SO_2 OR Asia = 1.044, 95%CI [0.954,1.142], P = .352 • Exposure to SO_2 OR overall = 1.085, 95%CI [1.013,1.163], P = .020)

| Lin et al,[35] 2021 | Effect of particulate matter exposure on the prevalence of allergic rhinitis in children: a systematic review and meta-analysis. | n = 217,396 | • Exposure to PM_{10} (OR Europe = 1.190, 95%CI [1.092,1.297], P = .000
• Exposure to PM_{10} OR Asia = 1.075, 95%CI [0.995,1.161], P = .066
• Exposure to PM_{10} OR overall = 1.125, 95%CI [1.062,1.191], P = .000)
• Exposure to $PM_{2.5}$ (OR Europe = 1.195, 95%CI [1.050,1.360], P = .007
• Exposure to $PM_{2.5}$ OR Asia = 1.163, 95%CI [1.074,1.260], P = .000
• Exposure to $PM_{2.5}$ OR overall = 1.172, 95%CI [1.095,1.254], P = .000).
• Exposed to air pollution probable is a risk of prevalence of childhood AR.
• The prevalence of AR will be increased when exposed to NO_2, SO_2, PM_{10} and $PM_{2.5}$, but maybe the relationship between SO_2/PM_{10} and prevalence of AR are not closely in Asia. |
| Zhou et al,[40] 2021 | Maternal tobacco exposure during pregnancy and allergic rhinitis in offspring: a systematic review and meta-analysis. | n = 1,149,879 | • An association between exposure to PM and the risk of childhood AR.
• The PM exposure is a risk factor for AR among children, whether PM_{10} or $PM_{2.5}$.
• $PM_{2.5}$ could affect the relation more than PM_{10}
• Maternal smoking exposure during pregnancy would increase the risk of allergic rhinitis in offspring (OR = 1.13,95%CI:1.02–1.26), especially maternal passive smoking during pregnancy (OR = 1.39,95%CI:1.05–1.84).
• Subgroup analysis showed that maternal active smoking during pregnancy was only significantly associated with offspring allergic rhinitis in cross-sectional studies (OR = 1.24,95%CI:1.07–1.45) and study done in America study (OR = 1.22,95%CI:1.05–1.42). |

(continued on next page)

Table 1
(continued)

Author/Year	Title	Number of Participants	Results/Conclusion
Gruzieva et al,[48] 2014	Meta-analysis of air pollution exposure association with allergic sensitization in European birth cohorts.	n= >6500	• Prevalence of sensitization to any common allergen within the 5 cohorts ranged between 24.1% and 40.4% at the age of 4–6 years. • Prevalence of sensitization to any common allergen within the 5 cohorts ranged between 34.8% and 47.9% at the age of 8–10 years. • Overall, air pollution exposure was not associated with sensitization to any common allergen, with odds ratios ranging from 0.94 (95%CI, 0.63–1.40) for a 1×10^{-5} m^{-1} increase in measurement of the blackness of PM$_{2.5}$ filters to 1.26 (95%CI, 0.90–1.77) for a 5 μg/m^3 increase in PM2.5 exposure at birth address. • Further analyses did not provide consistent evidence for a modification of the air pollution effects by sex, family history of atopy, or moving status. • No clear associations between air pollution exposure and development of allergic sensitization in children up to 10 years of age were revealed.

Table 2
Asthma and air pollution

Author/Year	Title	Number of Participants	Results/Conclusion
Skaaby et al,[39] 2017	Investigating the causal effect of smoking on hay fever and asthma: a Mendelian randomization meta-analysis in the CARTA consortium.	n = 231,020	• Observational analyses showed that current vs never smokers had lower risk of hay fever (odds ratio (OR) = 0.68, 95% confidence interval (CI): 0.61, 0.76; $P < 0.001$) and allergic sensitization (OR = 0.74, 95% CI: 0.64, 0.86; $P < 0.001$), but similar asthma risk (OR = 1.00, 95% CI: 0.91, 1.09; $P = 0.967$). • Mendelian randomization analyses in current smokers showed a slightly lower risk of hay fever (OR = 0.958, 95% CI: 0.920, 0.998; $P = 0.041$), a lower risk of allergic sensitization (OR = 0.92, 95% CI: 0.84, 1.02; $P = 0.117$), but higher risk of asthma (OR = 1.06, 95% CI: 1.01, 1.11; $P = 0.020$) per smoking-increasing allele. • Results suggest that smoking may be causally related to a higher risk of asthma and a slightly lower risk of hay fever. However, the adverse events associated with smoking limit its clinical significance.
Khreis et al,[41] 2017	Exposure to traffic-related air pollution and risk of development of childhood asthma: A systematic review and meta-analysis.	n = 1,292,255	• The overall random-effects risk estimates (95% CI) were: • 1.08 (1.03, 1.14) per 0.5×10^{-5} m^{-1} black carbon (BC) • 1.05 (1.02, 1.07) per 4 µg/m^3 nitrogen dioxide (NO_2) • 1.48 (0.89, 2.45) per 30 µg/m^3 nitrogen oxides (NO_x) • 1.03 (1.01, 1.05) per 1 µg/m^3 Particulate Matter < 2.5 µm in diameter ($PM_{2.5}$) • 1.05 (1.02, 1.08) per 2 µg/m^3 Particulate Matter < 10 µm in diameter (PM_{10}) • Sensitivity analyses supported these findings. • Across the main analysis and age-specific analysis: • the least heterogeneity was seen for the BC estimates • some heterogeneity for the $PM_{2.5}$ and PM_{10} estimates • the most heterogeneity for the NO_2 and NO_x estimates.

(continued on next page)

Table 2
(continued)

Author/Year	Title	Number of Participants	Results/Conclusion
Han et al,[42] 2020	Traffic-related organic and inorganic air pollution and risk of development of childhood asthma: A meta-analysis.	n = 1,310,479	• TRAP increased the risk of asthma among children: • $PM_{2.5}$ (meta-OR = 1.07, 95% CI:1.00–1.13) • NO_2 (meta-OR = 1.11, 95% CI:1.06–1.17) • Benzene (meta-OR: 1.21, 95% CI:1.13–1.29) • TVOC (meta-OR:1.06, 95% CI: 1.03–1.10). • Sensitivity analyses supported these findings. • Regional analysis showed that ORs of inorganic TRAP ($PM_{2.5}$ and NO_2) on the risk of childhood asthma were significantly higher in Asia than those in Europe and North America.
Thacher et al,[45] 2018	Maternal smoking during pregnancy and early childhood and development of asthma and rhinoconjunctivitis - a MeDALL project.	n = 10,860	• Any maternal smoking during pregnancy tended to be associated with an increased odds of prevalent asthma [adjusted odds ratio (aOR) = 1.19 (95% CI: 0.98, 1.43)], but not prevalent rhinoconjunctivitis [aOR = 1.05 (95% CI: 0.90, 1.22)], during childhood and adolescence. • In analyses with phenotypes related to age of onset and persistence of disease, any maternal smoking during pregnancy was associated with early transient asthma [aOR = 1.79 (95% CI: 1.14, 2.83)]. • Maternal smoking of ≥10 cigarettes/day during pregnancy was associated with persistent asthma [aOR = 1.66 (95% CI: 1.29, 2.15)] and persistent rhinoconjunctivitis [aOR = 1.55 (95% CI, 1.09, 2.20)]. • Tobacco smoke exposure during fetal life, infancy, childhood, and adolescence was not associated with adolescent-onset asthma or rhinoconjunctivitis. • Children with high early-life exposure were more likely than unexposed children to have early transient and persistent asthma and persistent rhinoconjunctivitis.

| Orellano et al,[47] 2017 | Effect of outdoor air pollution on asthma exacerbations in children and adults: Systematic review and multilevel meta-analysis. | n = 267,413 | • All pollutants except SO_2 and PM_{10} showed a significant association with asthma exacerbations:
• NO_2: 1.024; 95% CI: 1.005,1.043,
• SO_2: 1.039; 95% CI: 0.988,1.094),
• PM_{10}: 1.024; 95% CI: 0.995,1.053,
• $PM_{2.5}$: 1.028; 95% CI: 1.009,1.047,
• CO: 1.045; 95% CI: 1.005,1.086,
• O_3: 1.032; 95% CI: 1.005,1.060.
• In children, the association was significant for NO_2, SO_2 and $PM_{2.5}$. |

emergency department visits and admission.[46] This is further supported by findings of a systematic review and meta-analysis by Orellano and colleagues (as illustrated in **Table 2**) that demonstrated that the association between asthma exacerbation and air pollutants, especially NO_2 and $PM_{2.5}$ in the children population was significant.[47]

SUMMARY

Air quality has an important global impact on many health conditions and outcomes. This review demonstrates the effect it has on the upper and lower airway system in terms of its role as an environmental factor in the pathogenesis and outcomes of allergic rhinitis and asthma. Air pollution has a significant effect on the health and well-being of children in both the developing and the developed world and recognition and awareness to this issue on the global perspective needs to be continued and reinforced to help mitigate the adverse health effects due to its exposure.

CLINICS CARE POINTS

- Air pollution is a serious global issue with far reaching impact on human health including pathogenesis and exacerbation of chronic airway and sinonasal disease.
- Traffic-related airbone pollution (TRAP) can be associated with development of asthma and allergic rhinitis from very early exposure in the prenatal period and the early years of childhood.
- TRAP and Indoor air pollution such as smoking has been associated with poorer asthma outcomes, earlier onset and more severe exacerbations

FUNDING

Ramanathan- NIH grant funding R01AI143731.

REFERENCES

1. WHO global air quality guidelines: particulate matter (PM2.5 and PM10), ozone, nitrogen dioxide, sulfur dioxide and carbon monoxide. Geneva: World Health Organization; 2021.
2. What Is Air Pollution? https://www.who.int/docs/default-source/searo/wsh-och-searo/what-is-air-pollution-2019.pdf?sfvrsn=6dcc13ee_2.
3. US EPA. Criteria Air Pollutants | US EPA. US EPA. Published January 29, 2019. https://www.epa.gov/criteria-air-pollutants.
4. Orellano P, Reynoso J, Quaranta N, et al. Short-term exposure to particulate matter (PM10 and PM2.5), nitrogen dioxide (NO2), and ozone (O3) and all-cause and cause-specific mortality: Systematic review and meta-analysis. Environ Int 2020; 142:105876.
5. Tiotiu AI, Novakova P, Nedeva D, et al. Impact of air pollution on asthma outcomes. Int J Environ Res Public Health 2020;17(17):6212.
6. Sompornrattanaphan M, Thongngarm T, Ratanawatkul P, et al. The contribution of particulate matter to respiratory allergy. Asian Pac J Allergy Immunol 2020;38(1): 19–28.
7. Keswani A, Akselrod H, Anenberg SC. Health and clinical impacts of air pollution and linkages with climate change. NEJM Evidence 2022;1(7). https://doi.org/10.1056/evidra2200068.

8. Kelly FJ, Fussell JC. Size, source and chemical composition as determinants of toxicity attributable to ambient particulate matter. Atmos Environ 2012;60:504–26.
9. Thurston GD, Balmes JR, Garcia E, et al. Outdoor air pollution and new-onset airway disease: An official american thoracic society workshop report. Annals of the American Thoracic Society 2020;17:387–98. American Thoracic Society.
10. Lindgren A, Stroh E, Montnémery P, et al. Traffic-related air pollution associated with prevalence of asthma and COPD/chronic bronchitis. a cross-sectional study in Southern Sweden. Int J Health Geogr 2009;8(1). https://doi.org/10.1186/1476-072X-8-2.
11. London NR, Lina I, Ramanathan M. Aeroallergens, air pollutants, and chronic rhinitis and rhinosinusitis. World J Otorhinolaryngol Head Neck Surg 2018;4(3): 209–15.
12. Liu L, Ma J, Peng S, et al. Prenatal and early-life exposure to traffic-related air pollution and allergic rhinitis in children: A systematic literature review. PLoS One 2023;18(4):e0284625.
13. Rosario Filho NA, Satoris RA, Scala WR. Allergic rhinitis aggravated by air pollutants in Latin America: A systematic review. World Allergy Organ J 2021;14(8): 100574.
14. Gehring U, Gruzieva O, Agius RM, et al. Air pollution exposure and lung function in children: the ESCAPE project. Environ Health Perspect 2013;121(11–12): 1357–64.
15. Khreis H, Kelly C, Tate J, et al. Exposure to traffic-related air pollution and risk of development of childhood asthma: A systematic review and meta-analysis. Environ Int 2017;100:1–31.
16. Fukuoka A, Matsushita K, Morikawa T, et al. Diesel exhaust particles exacerbate allergic rhinitis in mice by disrupting the nasal epithelial barrier. Clin Exp Allergy 2016;46(1):142–52.
17. Kim JA, Cho JH, Park IH, et al. Diesel exhaust particles upregulate interleukins IL-6 and IL-8 in nasal fibroblasts. PLoS One 2016;11(6). https://doi.org/10.1371/journal.pone.0157058.
18. Breysse PN, Diette GB, Matsui EC, et al. Indoor air pollution and asthma in children. Proc Am Thorac Soc 2010;7(2):102–6.
19. Hulin M, Simoni M, Viegi G, et al. Respiratory health and indoor air pollutants based on quantitative exposure assessments. Eur Respir J 2012;40(4):1033–45.
20. Christensen DN, Franks ZG, McCrary HC, et al. A systematic review of the association between cigarette smoke exposure and chronic rhinosinusitis. Otolaryngol Head Neck Surg 2018;158(5):801–16.
21. Mulligan JK, Nagel W, O'Connell BP, et al. Cigarette smoke exposure is associated with vitamin D3 deficiencies in patients with chronic rhinosinusitis. J Allergy Clin Immunol 2014;134(2):342–9.e1.
22. Lee HS, Kim J. Cigarette smoke inhibits nasal airway epithelial cell growth and survival. Int Forum Allergy Rhinol 2013;3(3):188–92.
23. Cohen NA, Zhang S, Sharp DB, et al. Cigarette smoke condensate inhibits transepithelial chloride transport and ciliary beat frequency. Laryngoscope 2009; 119(11):2269–74.
24. Eguiluz-Gracia I, Mathioudakis AG, Bartel S, et al. The need for clean air: The way air pollution and climate change affect allergic rhinitis and asthma. Allergy 2020; 75(9):2170–84.
25. Wise SK, Damask C, Roland LT, et al. International consensus statement on allergy and rhinology: Allergic rhinitis - 2023. Int Forum Allergy Rhinol 2023; 13(4):293–859.

26. Diaz-Sanchez D, Tsien A, Casillas A, et al. Enhanced nasal cytokine production in human beings after in vivo challenge with diesel exhaust particles. J Allergy Clin Immunol 1996;98(1):114–23.

27. Diaz-Sanchez D, Garcia MP, Wang M, et al. Nasal challenge with diesel exhaust particles can induce sensitization to a neoallergen in the human mucosa. J Allergy Clin Immunol 1999;104(6):1183–8.

28. Ramanathan M Jr, London NR Jr, Tharakan A, et al. Airborne particulate matter induces nonallergic eosinophilic sinonasal inflammation in mice. Am J Respir Cell Mol Biol 2017;57(1):59–65.

29. Kim BJ, Kwon JW, Seo JH, et al. Association of ozone exposure with asthma, allergic rhinitis, and allergic sensitization. Ann Allergy Asthma Immunol 2011; 107(3):214–9.e1.

30. Gehring U, Wijga AH, Hoek G, et al. Exposure to air pollution and development of asthma and rhinoconjunctivitis throughout childhood and adolescence: a population-based birth cohort study. Lancet Respir Med 2015;3(12):933–42.

31. Franks ZG, London NR, Lee SE, et al. Long-term particulate matter exposure is associated with the development of nonallergic rhinitis: a case-control study. Int Forum Allergy Rhinol 2023;13(6):1042–5.

32. Li S, Wu W, Wang G, et al. Association between exposure to air pollution and risk of allergic rhinitis: A systematic review and meta-analysis. Environ Res 2022;205: 112472.

33. Zou QY, Shen Y, Ke X, et al. Exposure to air pollution and risk of prevalence of childhood allergic rhinitis: A meta-analysis. Int J Pediatr Otorhinolaryngol 2018; 112:82–90.

34. Teng B, Zhang X, Yi C, et al. The association between ambient air pollution and allergic rhinitis: further epidemiological evidence from Changchun, Northeastern China. Int J Environ Res Public Health 2017;14(3):226.

35. Lin L, Li T, Sun M, et al. Effect of particulate matter exposure on the prevalence of allergic rhinitis in children: A systematic review and meta-analysis. Chemosphere 2021;268:128841.

36. Chung HY, Hsieh CJ, Tseng CC, et al. Association between the first occurrence of allergic rhinitis in preschool children and air pollution in Taiwan. Int J Environ Res Public Health 2016;13(3):268.

37. Kim HH, Lee CS, Yu SD, et al. Near-road exposure and impact of air pollution on allergic diseases in elementary school children: a cross-sectional study. Yonsei Med J 2016;57(3):698–713.

38. Liu W, Huang C, Hu Y, et al. Associations of gestational and early life exposures to ambient air pollution with childhood respiratory diseases in Shanghai, China: A retrospective cohort study. Environ Int 2016;92-93:284–93.

39. Skaaby T, Taylor AE, Thuesen BH, et al. Estimating the causal effect of body mass index on hay fever, asthma and lung function using Mendelian randomization. Allergy 2018;73(1):153–64.

40. Zhou Y, Chen J, Dong Y, et al. Maternal tobacco exposure during pregnancy and allergic rhinitis in offspring: A systematic review and meta-analysis. Medicine (Baltim) 2021;100(34):e26986.

41. Khreis H, Kelly C, Tate J, et al. Exposure to traffic-related air pollution and risk of development of childhood asthma: a systematic review and meta-analysis. Environ Int 2017;100:1–31.

42. Han K, Ran Z, Wang X, et al. Traffic-related organic and inorganic air pollution and risk of development of childhood asthma: a meta-analysis. Environ Res 2021;194:110493.

43. Lau N, Norman A, Smith MJ, et al. Association between traffic related air pollution and the development of asthma phenotypes in children: a systematic review. Int J Chronic Dis 2018;2018:4047386.
44. Chen G, Zhou H, He G, et al. Effect of early-life exposure to $PM_{2.5}$ on childhood asthma/wheezing: a birth cohort study. Pediatr Allergy Immunol 2022;33(6). https://doi.org/10.1111/pai.13822.
45. Thacher JD, Gehring U, Gruzieva O, et al. Maternal smoking during pregnancy and early childhood and development of asthma and rhinoconjunctivitis - a MeD-ALL Project. Environ Health Perspect 2018;126(4):047005.
46. Li S, Batterman S, Wasilevich E, et al. Association of daily asthma emergency department visits and hospital admissions with ambient air pollutants among the pediatric Medicaid population in Detroit: time-series and time-stratified case-crossover analyses with threshold effects. Environ Res 2011;111(8): 1137–47.
47. Orellano P, Quaranta N, Reynoso J, et al. Effect of outdoor air pollution on asthma exacerbations in children and adults: systematic review and multilevel meta-analysis. PLoS One 2017;12(3):e0174050.
48. Gruzieva O, Gehring U, Aalberse R, et al. Meta-analysis of air pollution exposure association with allergic sensitization in European birth cohorts. J Allergy Clin Immunol 2014;133(3):767.

How Does Climate Change Affect the Upper Airway?

Jean Kim, MD, PhD[a,b,1,*], Benjamin Zaitchik, PhD[c,1],
Darryn Waugh, PhD[d,1]

KEYWORDS

- Climate change • Anthropogenic activity • Allergic rhinitis • Air pollution • $PM_{2.5}$
- Allergic fungal rhinosinusitis • Mold • Social determinants of health

KEY POINTS

- The prevalence of allergic rhinitis, chronic rhinosinusitis, and allergic fungal rhinosinusitis is increasing at an accelerated rate.
- Climate change is shifting ecological zones and seasons, increasing weather extremes, and altering regional atmospheric and environmental conditions.
- These climate factors can promote conditions for allergen growth, air pollution, and fungal growth, thereby promoting the increased prevalence of upper airway diseases.

INCREASED PREVALENCE OF AIRWAY DISEASE

There have been substantial increases in the prevalence of airway diseases during the last few decades. For example, there has been a worldwide increase in the prevalence of reported allergic rhinitis to an average of almost 30% of the world's population during the past 50 years with increases in Finland (0.6%–8.88%), Sweden (21%–31%), the United Kingdom (5.8%–19.9%), Northern Europe (19.7%–24.7%), Italy (16.2%–37.4%), South Korea (13.5%–17.1%), and Western Australia (21.9%–46.7%).[1] There are also documented increases in severe forms of chronic rhinosinusitis, such as allergic fungal rhinosinusitis (AFRS).[2] This form presents as one of the more common manifestations of upper airway fungal disease in both immunocompetent and immunocompromised individuals. Specifically, a recent review of AFRS in 35 urban cities from 5 continents demonstrated an increased prevalence seen in regions of higher

[a] Department of Otolaryngology-Head and Neck Surgery, Johns Hopkins University School of Medicine, Baltimore, USA; [b] Department of Medicine, Allergy and Clinical Immunology, Johns Hopkins University School of Medicine, Baltimore, USA; [c] Department of Earth and Planetary Sciences, Kennedy Krieger School of Arts and Sciences, Johns Hopkins University, 3400 N Charles Street, Olin Hall 301, Baltimore, MD 21218, USA; [d] Department of Earth and Planetary Sciences, Kennedy Krieger School of Arts and Sciences, Johns Hopkins University, 3400 N Charles Street, Olin Hall 320, Baltimore, MD 21218, USA
[1] All authors contributed equally.
* Corresponding author. Johns Hopkins Asthma and Allergy Center, Johns Hopkins Bayview Medical Center, 5501 Hopkins Bayview Circle, Rm 5A32, Baltimore, MD 21224.
E-mail address: jeankim@jhmi.edu

Otolaryngol Clin N Am 57 (2024) 309–317
https://doi.org/10.1016/j.otc.2023.09.008
0030-6665/24/© 2023 Elsevier Inc. All rights reserved.

oto.theclinics.com

temperatures, namely in subtropical areas.[2] In the United States, a higher incidence of AFRS is found along the Mississippi river basin and in the south-central part of the United States, where the presence of high humidity correlates strongly with the prevalence of disease.[3] This subtype of chronic rhinosinusitis is characterized by eosinophilic rich mucous and immunoglobulin E (IgE)-mediated type-1 hypersensitivity to fungal antigens in patients. Typical radiographic findings include paranasal sinus opacification with heterogeneous intrasinus densities and demineralization of sinus walls with bony expansion/erosion, often requiring timely surgical intervention.[4] Thus, the implication for increasing prevalence of AFRS will lead to increase in need for timely medical and advanced surgical treatment. There has also been an increased prevalence of other respiratory diseases. For example, a 25-year population study from Italy showed that the prevalence of asthma attacks more than doubled (from 3.4% to 7%) and chronic obstructive pulmonary disease almost tripled (from 2.1% to 6.8%).[5] A likely contributor to the above increases in disease prevalence is the changing climate.

GLOBAL WARMING DUE TO HUMAN ACTIVITY

Global temperatures have been increasing at a rate that Earth has not seen for thousands of years or longer, with human (or anthropogenic) activity as the dominant cause of this increase[6] (**Fig. 1**). This fact is documented in a massive body of climate science literature, which is regularly assessed by the Intergovernmental Panel on Climate Change (IPCC) to capture the state of scientific understanding.[7] The burning of fossil fuels, including coal, natural gas, and petroleum, in combination with loss of natural areas such as forests and wildlife habitats, has increased the concentrations of the greenhouse gases carbon dioxide, methane, and nitrous oxide in the atmosphere. These gases absorb and reemit thermal radiation that would otherwise escape more easily to outer space. This results in a warming of Earth's lower atmosphere and an increase in average land surface and ocean temperatures. Global warming, in turn, results in changes in other physical, chemical and biological properties within the climate system. The increased temperature increases the ability of the atmosphere to hold water, leading to an increase in absolute atmospheric humidity. Global warming is also associated with increases in frequency and severity of extreme events,

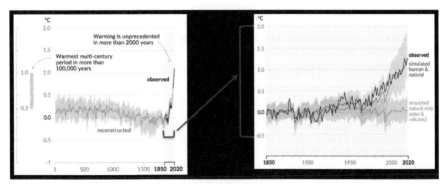

Fig. 1. Global Warming: Past and Future. Temperature changes on earth's atmospheric temperature in degree Celsius from year 1 AD to present (left panel). Changes in temperature due to human activity from the year 1850 to present (right panel). (Lee H, Romero J, et al. IPCC, 2023: Climate Change 2023: Synthesis Report. A Report of the Intergovernmental Panel on Climate Change. Contribution of Working Groups I, II and III to the Sixth Assessment Report of the Intergovernmental Panel on Climate. 2023: Geneva, Switzerland. p. In press. (http://www.ipcc.ch))

including heat waves, heavy rainfall, and droughts. There are also changes in characteristics of weather systems, associated movement of air, and changes in surface pressure.

As presented in later discussion, these changes in weather and climate have consequences for the prevalence of allergy-driven diseases, through changes in pollen, mold, and air pollution (**Fig. 2**).

CLIMATE CHANGE AND POLLEN GROWTH, SPREAD, AND POTENCY

The changes in climate have an effect on increasing pollen, which is known to directly drive prevalence of allergic rhinitis and allergic asthma. In certain vulnerable ecologic regions, increased heat and precipitation can result in increased pollen growth, whereas changes in weather patterns can promote the spread of pollen. In addition, the increase in atmospheric carbon dioxide has a "fertilizing" effect for many plants, accelerating their growth rate and increasing pollen production. Thus, climate change can offer physical conditions that both increase pollen production and alter the geography of its production and transport.

During the past 52 years, the length of freeze-free plant growing season has increased throughout the United States, with increases of around 3 weeks to more than 3 months.[8] This has resulted in the extension of the pollen season. During the past 30 years (from 1990 to 2018), there has been an extension across North America, with largest increases in Texas and the Midwest US .[9] In most of the United States, this increase in length includes an earlier start date to the pollen season.[9] Pollens belts have not only increased in size but have also migrated northward.[10] Plants that used to thrive in certain endogenous locations are now more suitable to grow in

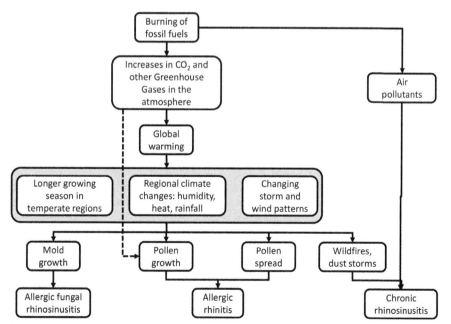

Fig. 2. Hypothesized pathways through which burning of fossil fuels and associated climate change can affect AFRS, allergic rhinitis, and chronic rhinosinusitis. Elevated CO_2 in the atmosphere influences pollen growth both through climate impacts and through CO_2 fertilization that affects growth and pollen production in some species (dashed *line*).

more northern locations. For example, North American allergenic species such as oak and hickory have increased at the expense of less allergenic pine and fir.[10]

The increase in atmospheric carbon dioxide that is a major cause of climate change also has its own direct influences on allergenic species. For example, Wayne and colleagues grew ragweed plants in both ambient (350 μL/L) JK and twice ambient (700 μL/L) JK carbon dioxide levels.[11] They observed that both the size of the ragweed plant and the ability of the plant to produce pollen were increased by 63% and 61%, respectively.[11] Furthermore, not only does climate change induce more pollen growth but also the pollen-induced plant seems to exhibit greater potency in its ability to stimulate an allergic inflammatory response. In a study by Rauer and colleagues, pollen produced by ragweed plants grown under elevated CO_2 elicited a stronger inflammatory response in a mouse model of allergic asthma, with potentiation of allergen-induced infiltration of lymphocytes, neutrophils, eosinophils from mouse lung tissue and greater induction of serum IgE.[12] In addition, in vitro exposure of human nasal epithelial cells grown in coculture with human dendritic cells to ragweed grown under elevated CO_2 resulted in increased cytokine tumor necrosis factor and decreased interleukin-10 production from dendritic cells.[12] These studies provide direct evidence of the ability of climate factors to induce allergic inflammation with greater intensity and potency.

CLIMATE CHANGE AND AIR POLLUTION

Poor air quality is well known to have a significant influence on airway diseases. The increase in atmospheric particulate matter less than 2.5 μm in diameter ($PM_{2.5}$) along with increases in greenhouse gases, nitrogen dioxide, and ozone has been shown to exacerbate chronic rhinosinusitis.[13-16] Of particular importance are changes in the concentration of suspended solid or liquid particles in the atmosphere, referred to as particulate matter (PM). $PM_{2.5}$ is about 25 times smaller than a diameter of human hair or approximately one-quarter the size of a typical allergen.[17,18] These particles reduce atmosphere visibility and can easily be inhaled into the airways, resulting in a range of negative health impacts, including asthma,[19-21] COPD,[22] and chronic rhinosinusitis.

PM has a wide range of sources, including power generation from coal and natural gas, automotive combustion, dust storms, and wildfires. As a result, human activities that have increased fossil fuel burning directly increase the concentration of $PM_{2.5}$. These activities also cause global warming and changes in weather and regional climate that are associated with increased wildfire risk[23-25] and increased droughts and dust[26] in many regions (see **Fig. 2**). Wildfires in the United States more than doubled during the past 40 years, foreboding the potential for more wildfire activity in the future. A very recent example of influences of wildfires is the movement of smoke and PM from Canadian wildfires in June 2023 (**Fig. 3**).[27] During 5th to 10th of June, the plume of smoke from these fires moved over the US east coast and the air quality over New York City and Baltimore reached unhealthy and dangerous levels (**Fig. 4**).[27,28] In contrast, Chicago was unaffected by the movement of wild fire smoke, and experienced no increase in air quality index (AQI).[28]

CLIMATE CHANGE AND FUNGAL GROWTH

Climate change has the ability to promote mold growth and survival, which can increase the prevalence of AFRS. Mold is fungus that forms in damp and decaying organic matter, which is found throughout all seasons and found both indoor and outdoor environments. Climate change leads to increased heavy rainfall events that

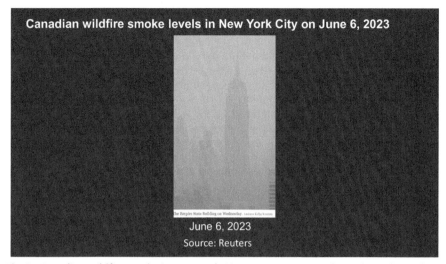

Fig. 3. Canadian wildfire smoke in New York City on June 6, 2023. Photo shows haze along Manhattan skyline. Source from New York Times.[27]

provide the damp environment, which promotes mold growth and survival. Climate change also leads to increased droughts in many regions, and these events promote decay of organic matter to provide food for mold.[29]

Mold is one of the most common and potent allergens. Many other species of fungi also serve as direct human pathogens. In addition, fungus can also have devastating effects on food plants. Although viral and bacterial disease have recently received much attention in biomedical research during the pandemic, it is important to recognize that fungi have the potential to produce great threats.[30] Fungi can live saprophytically,

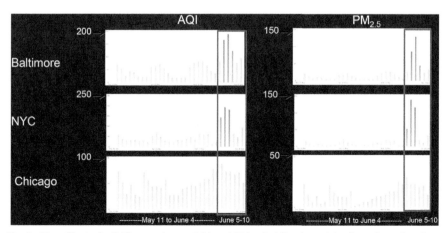

Fig. 4. The effect of wildfire smoke on AQI and $PM_{2.5}$ in US urban cities from June 5 to June 10, 2023. AQI < 100 or $PM_{2.5}$ < 12 $\mu g/m^3$ are acceptable levels. Pink square highlights values during the Canadian wildfire in Baltimore, New York City, and Chicago. (Air quality index (AQI) and PM2.5 air pollution in USA. 2023 July 21, 2023 [cited 2023 June 10. 2023]; Interactive map of air quality index and PM2.5 levels].Available from: https://www.iqair.com/us/usa.)

producing large quantities of spores that can be inhaled into the airways. Currently, there are no vaccines available for the treatment of fungal pathogens, and the number of antifungal agents is extremely limited. New fungal species have emerged to cause significant outbreaks that seem related to climate change. These species are now benefiting from warmer environments, resulting in increased influences on human, animal, and plant health.[30] *Batrachochytrium dendrobatidis* is an amphibian pathogen found in the tropics that is now spreading to North America, South America, and Australia. *Cryptococcus deuterogattii* is a human lung pathogen that is growing in Canada and the US Pacific northwest. This pathogen has the ability to spread hematologically from spores inhaled through the lungs to infect the nervous system. *Puccinia striiformis* (Rust fungus) is a wheat crop pathogen has adapted to growth in warmer temperatures and is spreading to United States and Australia. Fusarium head blight is another wheat crop pathogen, which has caused food insecurity in many areas of the world, including Asia, Canada, Europe, and South America[30,31] These data highlight the importance of understanding how environmental mold growth patterns are changing over time and the need for ongoing research in these areas.

UNIFIED AIRWAY RISKS IN A CHANGING CLIMATE

Understanding, preparing for, and responding to climate-associated airway risks require a holistic view of the factors that contribute to risk. In the fields of natural hazards and climate change, this view is frequently framed as a "risk propeller" (**Fig. 5**), in which risk is placed at the intersection of hazard, exposure, vulnerability, and response.[32,33] In this framing, the instigating climate *hazard*—an acute event such as a flood, or a persistent phenomenon such as a longer pollen season—results in *exposures* with potential health impacts. The magnitude and distribution of these impacts, however, depends

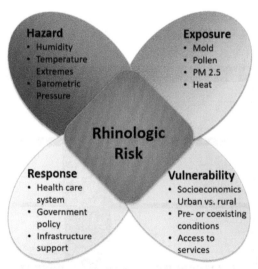

Fig. 5. Climate risk propeller. The "risk propeller" applied to rhinologic disease. The "risk propeller" is frequently used in IPCC Reports. Risk is understood to be a product of interactions between climate hazards, exposures related to factors that endanger people, vulnerabilities that predispose people or groups to adverse impacts, and responses that either mitigate or inadvertently exacerbate the risk of negative outcomes. (Kim J, et al. Climate change, the environment, and rhinologic disease. International Forum of Allergy & Rhinology, 2023. 13(5): p. 865 to 876.)

on the *vulnerability* of the exposed population. For example, risk factors for AFRS in the United States include being of African American descent, lower socioeconomic status, and male sex.[34] In many cases, health impacts are also mediated by the social and health system *responses* to the recognized risk.

Figure 5 is presented only as an indicative way in which the propeller framework can be applied to explore risk factors relevant to airway health outcomes. The same approach can be applied to any set of airway risks thought to be sensitive to climate conditions. Doing so can offer some clarity on the mechanism and magnitude of climate influence on a health impact of concern, and it can also point the way to potential interventions. Reducing a climate hazard, for example, may require large-scale climate change mitigation efforts or changes in land use and the design of the built environment. Reducing exposure might be achieved through behavioral recommendations, targeted building improvements, indoor environment controls, or other local interventions. Vulnerabilities may point to specific social or demographic dynamics that need to be addressed and that should be considered by caregivers seeing patients from more vulnerable groups. Improved response to an evolving climate-related health risk can be taken on through health systems, broader governmental policy initiatives, and the informed actions of health practitioners.

Placing potential climate-related risks to the unified airway in this systematic framework offers an opportunity to characterize interacting risk factors and to identify areas in need of further research. Framing climate-related risks in this way also offers pathways to action: a changing climate means changes in airway risks, and evidence has shown that this often means an increase in risk. However, there are many levers available to anticipate in order to combat these risks as they emerge.

CLINICS CARE POINTS

- Health-care providers should be alerted to the potential detrimental effect of climate change on upper airway disease.
- These factors include excessive heat, increased allergens including mold, and increased air pollution.
- Notably, the underserved population will be most vulnerable to these effects.
- Research and collaboration between health-care providers and other sectors of our society including government, industry, and academia is needed to address these global consequences to health.

DISCLOSURE

J. Kim has grant funding from Genentech Roche, United States and Glaxo Smith Kline (GSK), United Kingdom. All other authors declare no conflicts of interest.

REFERENCES

1. Savoure M, Bousquet J, Jaakkola JJK, et al. Worldwide prevalence of rhinitis in adults: A review of definitions and temporal evolution. Clin Transl Allergy 2022; 12(3):e12130.
2. AlQahtani A, Alim B, Almudhaibery F, et al. The Impact of Climatic, Socioeconomic, and Geographic Factors on the Prevalence of Allergic Fungal Rhinosinusitis: A Worldwide Ecological Study. Am J Rhinol Allergy 2022;36(4):423–31.

3. Ferguson BJ, Barnes L, Bernstein JM, et al. Geographic variation in allergic fungal rhinosinusitis. Otolaryngol Clin North Am 2000;33(2):441–9.
4. Kim J, Makary CA, Roland LT, et al. What is allergic fungal sinusitis: A call to action. International Forum of Allergy & Rhinology 2022;12(2):141–6.
5. Maio S, Baldacci S, Carrozzi L, et al. Respiratory symptoms/diseases prevalence is still increasing: a 25-yr population study. Respir Med 2016;110:58–65.
6. Lee H, Calvin K, Dasgupta D, et al. Climate Change 2023: Synthesis Report. A Report of the Intergovernmental Panel on Climate Change. In: Lee H, Romero J, editors. *Contribution of working groups I, II and III to the Sixth assessment Report of the intergovernmental panel on climate change*. 2023. Geneva, Switzerland.
7. Prasad, A.M., L.R. Iverson, S. Matthews, M. Peters, 2007-ongoing. A Climate Change Atlas for 134 Forest Tree Species of the Eastern United States database. 2007.
8. Ziska, L., J. Bell, and B. Lappe. Allergy Season: Earlier, Longer, and Worse. Climate Central July 17, 2023; Available from: https://www.climatecentral.org/climate-matters/allergy-season-earlier-longer-and-worse-2023.
9. Anderegg WRL, Abatzoglou JT, Anderegg LDL, et al. Anthropogenic climate change is worsening North American pollen seasons. Proceedings of the National Academy of Sciences of the United States of America 2021;118(7). e2013284118.
10. Staudt A, Glick P, Mizejewski D, et al. Extreme allergies and global warming. National Wildlife Federation; 2010.
11. Wayne P, Foster S, Connolly J, et al. Production of allergenic pollen by ragweed (Ambrosia artemisiifolia L.) is increased in CO2-enriched atmospheres. Ann Allergy Asthma Immunol 2002;88(3):279–82.
12. Rauer D, Gilles S, Wimmer M, et al. Ragweed plants grown under elevated CO2 levels produce pollen which elicit stronger allergic lung inflammation. Allergy 2021;76(6):1718–30.
13. McCormick JP, Lee JT. The Role of Airborne Pollutants in Chronic Rhinosinusitis. Current Treatment Options in Allergy 2021;8(4):314–23.
14. Ramanathan M Jr, London NR, Tharakan A, et al. Airborne Particulate Matter Induces Nonallergic Eosinophilic Sinonasal Inflammation in Mice. Am J Respir Cell Mol Biol 2017;57(1):59–65.
15. Zhang Z, Kamil RJ, London NR, et al. Long-Term Exposure to Particulate Matter Air Pollution and Chronic Rhinosinusitis in Nonallergic Patients. Am J Respir Crit Care Med 2021;204(7):859–62.
16. Patel TR, Tajudeen BA, Brown H, et al. Association of Air Pollutant Exposure and Sinonasal Histopathology Findings in Chronic Rhinosinusitis. Am J Rhinol Allergy 2021;35(6):761–7.
17. Agency EP. Climate change and children's health and well-being in the United States. U.S. Environmental Protection Agency; 2023.
18. Thangavel P, Park D, Lee YC. Recent Insights into Particulate Matter ($PM_{2.5}$)-Mediated Toxicity in Humans: An Overview. Int J Environ Res Public Health 2022;19(12):7511.
19. Guarnieri M, Balmes JR. Outdoor air pollution and asthma. Lancet 2014;383(9928):1581–92.
20. Liu K, Hua S, Song L. PM2.5 Exposure and Asthma Development: The Key Role of Oxidative Stress. Oxid Med Cell Longev 2022;2022:3618806.

21. Lu MX, Ding SR, Wang JY, et al. Acute effect of ambient air pollution on hospital outpatient cases of chronic sinusitis in Xinxiang, China. Ecotoxicology and Environmental Safety 2020;202.
22. Hansel NN, McCormack MC, Kim V. The Effects of Air Pollution and Temperature on COPD. COPD 2016;13(3):372–9.
23. Abatzoglou JT, Williams AP. Impact of anthropogenic climate change on wildfire across western US forests. Proc Natl Acad Sci USA 2016;113(42):11770–5.
24. Smith A, Jones M, Abatzoglou J, et al. Climate change increases the risk of wildfires. Critical Issues in Climate Change Science 2020.
25. Whitman E, Sherren K, Rapaport E. Increasing daily wildfire risk in the Acadian Forest Region of Nova Scotia, Canada, under future climate change. Reg Environ Change 2015;15(7):1447–59.
26. Achakulwisut P, Shen L, Mickley LJ. What Controls Springtime Fine Dust Variability in the Western United States? Investigating the 2002–2015 Increase in Fine Dust in the U.S. Southwest. J Geophys Res Atmos 2017;122(22):12449–67.
27. Dong M., Maksky, B., Gamio L., et al., Maps: Tracking Air Quality and Smoke From Wildfires, In: New York times, 2023, New York Times; New York, NY, USA.
28. Air quality index (AQI) and PM2.5 air pollution in USA. 2023 July 21, 2023 cited 2023 June 10. 2023; Interactive map of air quality index and PM2.5 levels. Available from: https://www.iqair.com/us/usa.
29. Touma D, Stevenson S, Swain DL, et al. Climate change increases risk of extreme rainfall following wildfire in the western United States. Sci Adv 2022;8(13): eabm0320.
30. Nnadi NE, Carter DA. Climate change and the emergence of fungal pathogens. PLoS Pathog 2021;17(4):e1009503.
31. Windels CE. Economic and Social Impacts of Fusarium Head Blight: Changing Farms and Rural Communities in the Northern Great Plains. Phytopathology® 2000;90(1):17–21.
32. Albertine JM, Manning WJ, DaCosta M, et al. Projected carbon dioxide to increase grass pollen and allergen exposure despite higher ozone levels. PLoS One 2014;9(11):e111712.
33. Simpson NP, Mach KJ, Constable A, et al. A framework for complex climate change risk assessment. One Earth 2021;4(4):489–501.
34. Orlandi R.R., Kingdom T.T., Smith T.L., et al., International consensus statement on allergy and rhinology: rhinosinusitis. *International Forum of Allergy & Rhinology.* 2021;11 (3), 2021, 211–739. https://doi.org/10.1002/alr.22741.

Allergic Rhinitis and Its Effect on Sleep

Jessica M.L. Pagel, AB[a], Jose L. Mattos, MD, MPH[b],*

KEYWORDS

- Allergic rhinitis • Sleep disturbance • Sleep-disordered breathing
- Obstructive sleep apnea

KEY POINTS

- Allergic rhinitis (AR) increases nasal obstruction and inflammatory mediators, decreasing quality of sleep and rapid eye movement (REM) while increasing sleep latency, sleep-disordered breathing, and obstructive sleep apnea.
- Patients with AR should be considered for sleep disorder evaluation. If evaluated using polysomnography, special consideration should be given to REM respiratory disturbance indices and respiratory effort-related arousals.
- Effective therapies for patients with AR and sleep disturbances include intranasal corticosteroids, non–central nervous system-penetrating antihistamines, and allergen immunotherapy. Inferior turbinate reduction may decrease sleep impairment in cases of AR and nasal obstruction.

INTRODUCTION

Although not considered a severely disabling disease, allergic rhinitis (AR), with a prevalence recently noted as high as 50.5%, has a large influence on quality of life in children and adults.[1] Sleep impairment, found in up to 66% of AR patients,[2] is a notable contributor. It may present as a patient's main complaint[3] because it leads to cognitive impairment, reduced productivity, and decreased quality of life.[4] The influence of sleep disturbances is such that, under ARIA (Allergic Rhinitis and its Impact on Asthma) guidelines, AR is categorized as moderate-to-severe if any sleep impairment is noted.[5]

DISCUSSION
Current Evidence

A close link exists between AR and sleep impairment. Liu and colleagues,[6] reviewing 27 observational studies, found patients with AR to have significantly higher odds of

[a] University of Virginia School of Medicine, 1340 Jefferson Park Avenue, Charlottesville, VA 22903, USA; [b] Department of Otolaryngology–Head and Neck Surgery, University of Virginia, 1 Hospital Drive, PO Box 800713, Charlottesville, VA 22908, USA
* Corresponding author.
E-mail address: jm6cb@uvahealth.org

Otolaryngol Clin N Am 57 (2024) 319–328
https://doi.org/10.1016/j.otc.2023.09.003
0030-6665/24/© 2023 Elsevier Inc. All rights reserved.

obstructive sleep apnea (OSA), sleep-disordered breathing (SDB), snoring, or nocturnal enuresis. Sleep dysfunction correlates with AR severity; patients with moderate-to-severe rhinitis reported increased nasal obstruction, increased awakenings, and decreased sleep quality compared with less symptomatic patients.[3,7] In addition, patients with seasonal AR have more frequent and longer apneic episodes during allergy season.[8]

The prevalence of AR in children is also high, with 31% reporting symptoms in a recent community study.[9] In pediatric studies, AR has been associated with SDB, restless sleep, night arousals, snoring, sleep routine problems, decreased rapid eye movement (REM) sleep, and nocturnal enuresis.[9–12]

Although Liu and colleagues[6] noted elevated odds of OSA and SDB, the relationship between AR and OSA is unclear. Studies of adults with AR have noted both elevated[13,14] and comparable OSA risk[15] with no influence on severity.[14] In children, a meta-analysis of 18 studies revealed a positive association between AR and SDB in most studies.[16] However, AR has no influence on the obstructive apnea-hypopnea index or apnea-hypopnea index (AHI) in children with SDB.[17]

The pathophysiology of how AR affects sleep is multifactorial (**Fig. 1**); however, one major factor is nasal obstruction, which itself is an independent risk factor for sleep impairment.[18] After allergen exposure, late-phase reaction congestion leads to dilated capacitance vessels, decreasing nasal diameter and causing obstruction.[18] This congestion in AR has been associated with increased episodes of apnea and microarousals in sleep.[19]

In addition, inflammatory cytokines, specifically interleukin (IL)-1β, IL-4, and IL-10, are released during allergic reactions and correlate with decreased REM sleep on polysomnography (PSG).[20] Histamine causes local vasodilation and mucus secretion, worsens nasal congestion and obstruction, and plays a central role in the sleep–wake cycle.[21] Cysteinyl leukotrienes also cause vasodilation and mucus secretion with more potent and longer effects.[22] Diurnal variation results in nasal obstruction[23] and inflammatory mediators[24] peaking in the early morning and is accompanied by an increase in parasympathetic tone at rest.[21]

Increased risk of OSA may be due to AR obstruction inhibiting nasal receptors and increasing airflow resistance.[8] OSA inflammatory mediators such as tumor necrosis factor, IL-1, and IL-6 then activate Th2 cells, increasing inflammation in the AR-primed environment.[25] This inflammation and obstruction may inhibit mechanoreceptors, decreasing activation of the nasal-ventilatory reflex[26] and muscle tone of the upper airway.[27]

Evaluation

Although a known side effect of AR pharmacologic treatment, fatigue should also be evaluated separately as a potential symptom of AR. Generally, any patient diagnosed with AR should be considered for a sleep evaluation. Commonly used tools in research include the Epworth Sleepiness Scale and Pittsburgh Sleep Quality Index. PSG may also be used, especially for concern of SDB. If used, providers should pay special attention to respiratory effort-related arousals and elevated REM respiratory disturbance indices (RDI) because in AR, PSG often displays normal AHI and RDI.[28] In patients with OSA and AR, providers should closely monitor initial tolerance of continuous airway pressure (CPAP) machines because it may act as a nonallergic trigger of nasal congestion.[29] Persistent nasal obstruction may lead to decreased CPAP compliance[30]; however, surgical correction can improve CPAP compliance and tolerance.[31]

In children with AR, providers should consider evaluation for SDB and OSA because AR is a predictive factor in underweight children.[32] Children with OSA

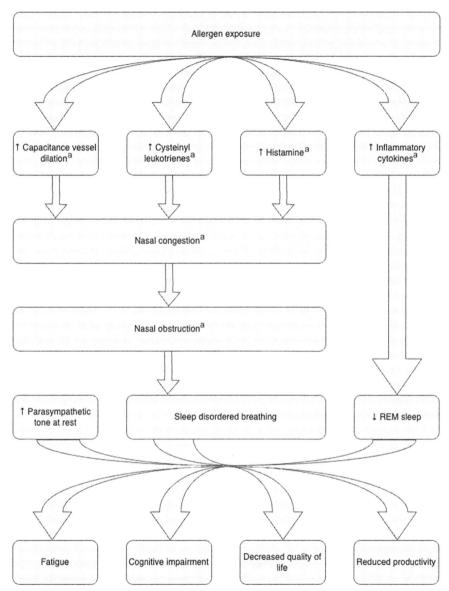

Fig. 1. Causes of sleep disturbance and fatigue in AR. [a]Exhibit diurnal version and worsen in the early morning.

should be evaluated for AR because it is a predictor of decreased quality of life after tonsillectomy.[33]

Therapeutic Options

Intranasal corticosteroids
Commonly used for AR, intranasal corticosteroids (INCS) target nasal obstruction, cytokines, and other inflammatory markers.[34] Craig and colleagues[35] first demonstrated

that nasal flunisolide could decrease nasal congestion, improve sleep quality, and decrease daytime sleepiness in patients with AR. Since then, other studies have noted similar self-reported improvement using budesonide and fluticasone.[36–39] In cohort studies and randomized controlled trials (RCTs), patients with OSA and AR using INCS had significantly decreased AHI events and lowered nasal airway resistance.[40–42]

INCS may benefit children with nasal obstruction and OSA but there is no research specific for AR.[43] In addition, studies are inconclusive on whether INCS suppresses pediatric growth; one RCT found a significantly decreased growth after 1 year of INCS,[44] whereas 2 others did not.[45,46]

Oral corticosteroids
No studies using oral corticosteroids have specifically evaluated AR or influence on sleep but previous research demonstrated dose-dependent symptomatic improvement in nasal obstruction with oral prednisolone[47] and betamethasone.[48] Nevertheless, given their unfavorable side effect profiles, including potential increases in sleep disturbances, oral corticosteroids are not used in treatment.

Antihistamines
Second-generation and third-generation H1 antihistamines, which block peripheral H1 receptors, are recommended by guidelines for their lack of central nervous system (CNS) effects and ability to improve sleep quality.[30,49] In comparisons of CNS-penetrating and nonpenetrating antihistamines for AR, only the latter significantly improved the self-reported sleep quality.[50] However, meta-analyses by Weiner and colleagues[51] concluded that INCS are more effective than second-generation antihistamines for sleep impairment.

Intranasal antihistamines, with selective peripheral H1 antagonism and rapid duration of action, may also be useful, having demonstrated self-reported sleep improvements in up to 85% of patients.[52]

Leukotriene receptor antagonists
In double-blinded RCTs, AR patients treated with montelukast have significantly improved sleep quality scores, with an equivalent effect on sleep as loratadine.[53,54] However, the addition of montelukast to INCS demonstrated no improvements in a 6-study meta-analysis.[55] In children, who may prefer its taste to other treatments, montelukast was found to significantly improve sleep quality compared with cetirizine (with both performing significantly better than placebo).[56]

Nasal decongestants
Although a small crossover trial demonstrated that xylometazoline improved transient AHI levels compared with placebo, it did not change self-reported sleep quality.[57] Decongestants are not recommended because they may cause insomnia, other stimulatory effects, and rhinitis medicamentosa.[21]

Allergen immunotherapy
Allergen immunotherapy (AIT), in the form of sublingual immunotherapy (SLIT) is recommended for adults with moderate-to-severe AR to grass pollen or house dust mites[58] or for inadequate relief from pharmacotherapy.[30,59,60] Patients with AR have reported significant improvements in sleep quality after 1 to 3 years of SLIT,[2,61] and an RCT by Jacobi and colleagues[62] demonstrated significantly improved subjective sleep quality from SLIT compared with placebo. In a meta-analysis of 26 double-blinded RCTs, subcutaneous immunotherapy improved AR symptoms significantly more than SLIT; however, sleep quality was not an evaluated factor.[63] A small retrospective analysis

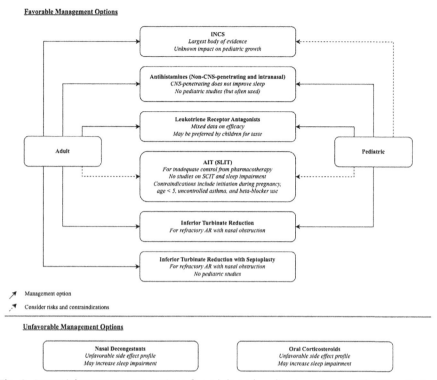

Fig. 2. Potential management options for adult and pediatric patients with AR suffering from sleep impairment.

of patients with AR undergoing SCIT evaluated for sleep disturbances but did not note any significant differences.[64] Most clinicians view AIT initiation during pregnancy, aged younger than 5 years, uncontrolled asthma, or systemic or topical beta-blocker usage as contraindications to AIT.[65]

Inferior turbinate reduction

Procedural management is offered for refractory cases of AR to address either structural or physiologic causes of symptoms. Procedures include viridian neurectomy, and posterior nasal nerve neurotomy or ablation, but only septoplasty and inferior turbinate reduction (ITR) have been evaluated for influence on sleep quality.

In adults with nasal obstruction and AR, snoring and sleep function were improved with ITR.[66–69] Kim and colleagues[70] observed a reduction in mean AHI and RDI in patients who underwent septoplasty and ITR with greater benefit for patients with AR and moderate-to-severe nasal obstruction. In children with AR and inferior turbinate (IT) hypertrophy, ITR alone may be of more use than adenotonsillectomy for snoring, nasal congestion, and AHI episodes.[71,72]

SUMMARY

AR affects sleep impairment, with multiple studies demonstrating an association between symptom severity and sleep disturbance. Currently, management of sleep impairment in AR consists of pharmacologic therapy, such as antihistamines and INCS, with AIT and ITR with or without septoplasty as options in specific cases (**Fig. 2**). In general, any patient with AR should be considered for sleep evaluation via screening questionnaires with a low bar for PSG evaluation given the relation among AR, sleep impairment, and SDB.

CLINICS CARE POINTS

- Although somnolence and sleep disturbance can occur as side effects of AR treatment, a careful evaluation should occur to separate pharmacologic side effects from AR symptomatology.

- Given its high prevalence and morbidity, patients with AR should be considered for sleep disorder evaluation. If evaluated by PSG, special consideration should be given to REM-RDI and respiratory effort-related arousals given often normal AHI and RDI.

- Effective therapies include INCS, non–CNS-penetrating antihistamines, and AIT (SLIT). AIT may be offered for inadequate pharmacologic control of sleep impairment in patients with AR.

- IT reduction strategies may improve sleep quality in cases of concomitant AR and nasal obstruction or IT hypertrophy.

DISCLOSURE

There are no other financial disclosures or conflicts of interest.

REFERENCES

1. Oliveira TB, Persigo ALK, Ferrazza CC, et al. Prevalence of asthma, allergic rhinitis and pollinosis in a city of Brazil: A monitoring study. Allergol Immunopathol 2020;48(6):537–44.
2. Romano M, James S, Farrington E, et al. The impact of perennial allergic rhinitis with/without allergic asthma on sleep, work and activity level. Allergy Asthma Clin Immunol 2019;15:81.
3. Leger D, Bonnefoy B, Pigearias B, et al. Poor sleep is highly associated with house dust mite allergic rhinitis in adults and children. Allergy Asthma Clin Immunol 2017;13:36.
4. Fineman SM. The burden of allergic rhinitis: beyond dollars and cents. Ann Allergy Asthma Immunol 2002;88(4 Suppl 1):2–7.
5. Bousquet J, Khaltaev N, Cruz AA, et al. Allergic rhinitis and its impact on asthma (ARIA) 2008 update (in collaboration with the World Health Organization, GA(2) LEN and AllerGen). Allergy 2008;63(Suppl 86):8–160.
6. Liu J, Zhang X, Zhao Y, et al. The association between allergic rhinitis and sleep: A systematic review and meta-analysis of observational studies. PLoS One 2020; 15(2):e0228533.
7. Colás C, Galera H, Añibarro B, et al. Disease severity impairs sleep quality in allergic rhinitis (The SOMNIAAR study). Clin Exp Allergy 2012;42(7):1080–7.
8. McNicholas WT, Tarlo S, Cole P, et al. Obstructive apneas during sleep in patients with seasonal allergic rhinitis. Am Rev Respir Dis 1982;126(4):625–8.
9. Sherrey J, Biggs S, Dorrian J, et al. Allergic disease, sleep problems, and psychological distress in children recruited from the general community. Ann Allergy Asthma Immunol 2022;129(3):366–72.
10. Wang Q, Guo Y, Wu X, et al. Effect of allergic rhinitis on sleep in children and the risk factors of an indoor environment. Sleep Breath 2022;26(3):1265–75.

11. Lai PH, Yang PS, Lai WY, et al. Allergic rhinitis and the associated risk of nocturnal enuresis in children: a population-based cohort study. Int Forum Allergy Rhinol 2018;8(11):1260–6.
12. Di Francesco RC, Alvarez J. Allergic rhinitis affects the duration of rapid eye movement sleep in children with sleep-disordered breathing without sleep apnea. Int Forum Allergy Rhinol 2016;6(5):465–71.
13. Chung C, Tsai M, Tsai Y, et al. Increased risk of sleep apnea in patients of allergic rhinitis - a nationwide population-based study. Dallas, TX: American Thoracic Society; 2019. Presented at.
14. Wongvilairat S, Assanasen P, Banhiran W, et al. The prevalence of high risk of obstructive sleep apnea in patients with allergic rhinitis. Asian Pac J Allergy Immunol 2022;40(3):205–9.
15. Pace A, Iannella G, Rossetti V, et al. Diagnosis of obstructive sleep apnea in patients with allergic and non-allergic rhinitis. Medicina (Kaunas) 2020;56(9):454.
16. Lin SY, TAN Melvin, Boss EF, et al. The association between allergic rhinitis and sleep-disordered breathing in children: a systematic review. Int Forum Allergy Rhinol 2013;3(6):504–9.
17. Liu J, Wu Y, Wu P, et al. Analysis of the impact of allergic rhinitis on the children with sleep disordered breathing. Int J Pediatr Otorhinolaryngol 2020;138:110380.
18. Corey JP, Houser SM, Ng BA. Nasal congestion: a review of its etiology, evaluation, and treatment. Ear Nose Throat J 2000;79(9):690–3, 696, 698 passim.
19. Craig TJ, Sherkat A, Safaee S. Congestion and sleep impairment in allergic rhinitis. Curr Allergy Asthma Rep 2010;10(2):113–21.
20. Krouse HJ, Davis JE, Krouse JH. Immune mediators in allergic rhinitis and sleep. Otolaryngol Head Neck Surg 2002;126(6):607–13.
21. Ferguson BJ. Influences of allergic rhinitis on sleep. Otolaryngol Head Neck Surg 2004;130(5):617–29.
22. Miadonna A, Tedeschi A, Leggieri E, et al. Behavior and clinical relevance of histamine and leukotrienes C4 and B4 in grass pollen-induced rhinitis. Am Rev Respir Dis 1987;136(2):357–62.
23. Reinberg A, Gervais P, Levi F, et al. Circadian and circannual rhythms of allergic rhinitis: an epidemiologic study involving chronobiologic methods. J Allergy Clin Immunol 1988;81(1):51–62.
24. Craig TJ, Ferguson BJ, Krouse JH. Sleep impairment in allergic rhinitis, rhinosinusitis, and nasal polyposis. Am J Otolaryngol 2008;29(3):209–17.
25. Tan S, Abdullah B. The association between obstructive sleep apnea and allergic rhinitis: current literature review. Curr Respir Med Rev 2021;17. 1-0.
26. McNicholas WT, Coffey M, Boyle T. Effects of nasal airflow on breathing during sleep in normal humans. Am Rev Respir Dis 1993;147(3):620–3.
27. Shintaro C, Park CS. Establishing a patent nasal passage in obstructive sleep apnea. Sleep Med Clin 2019;14(1):41–50.
28. Berson SR, Klimczak JA, Prezio EA, et al. House dust mite related allergic rhinitis and REM sleep disturbances. Am J Otolaryngol 2020;41(6):102709.
29. Skirko JR, James KT, Shusterman DJ, et al. Association of allergic rhinitis with change in nasal congestion in new continuous positive airway pressure users. JAMA Otolaryngol Head Neck Surg 2020;146(6):523–9.
30. Wise SK, Damask C, Roland LT, et al. International consensus statement on allergy and rhinology: Allergic rhinitis - 2023. Int Forum Allergy Rhinol 2023; 13(4):293–859.
31. Awad MI, Kacker A. Nasal obstruction considerations in sleep apnea. Otolaryngol Clin 2018;51(5):1003–9.

32. Johnson C, Leavitt T, Daram SP, et al. Obstructive sleep apnea in underweight children. Otolaryngol Head Neck Surg 2022;167(3):566–72.

33. Kim DK, Han DH. Impact of allergic rhinitis on quality of life after adenotonsillectomy for pediatric sleep-disordered breathing. Int Forum Allergy Rhinol 2015;5(8):741–6.

34. González-Núñez V, Valero AL, Mullol J. Impact of sleep as a specific marker of quality of life in allergic rhinitis. Curr Allergy Asthma Rep 2013;13(2):131–41.

35. Craig TJ, Teets S, Lehman EB, et al. Nasal congestion secondary to allergic rhinitis as a cause of sleep disturbance and daytime fatigue and the response to topical nasal corticosteroids. J Allergy Clin Immunol 1998;101(5):633–7.

36. Hughes K, Glass C, Ripchinski M, et al. Efficacy of the topical nasal steroid budesonide on improving sleep and daytime somnolence in patients with perennial allergic rhinitis. Allergy 2003;58(5):380–5.

37. Craig TJ, Hanks CD, Fisher LH. How do topical nasal corticosteroids improve sleep and daytime somnolence in allergic rhinitis? J Allergy Clin Immunol 2005;116(6):1264–6.

38. Gurevich F, Glass C, Davies M, et al. The effect of intranasal steroid budesonide on the congestion-related sleep disturbance and daytime somnolence in patients with perennial allergic rhinitis. Allergy Asthma Proc 2005;26(4):268–74.

39. Mansfield LE, Posey CR. Daytime sleepiness and cognitive performance improve in seasonal allergic rhinitis treated with intranasal fluticasone propionate. Allergy Asthma Proc 2007;28(2):226–9.

40. Kiely JL, Nolan P, McNicholas WT. Intranasal corticosteroid therapy for obstructive sleep apnoea in patients with co-existing rhinitis. Thorax 2004;59(1):50–5.

41. Acar M, Cingi C, Sakallioglu O, et al. The effects of mometasone furoate and desloratadine in obstructive sleep apnea syndrome patients with allergic rhinitis. Am J Rhinol Allergy 2013;27(4):e113–6.

42. Lavigne F, Petrof BJ, Johnson JR, et al. Effect of topical corticosteroids on allergic airway inflammation and disease severity in obstructive sleep apnoea. Clin Exp Allergy 2013;43(10):1124–33.

43. Brouillette RT, Manoukian JJ, Ducharme FM, et al. Efficacy of fluticasone nasal spray for pediatric obstructive sleep apnea. J Pediatr 2001;138(6):838–44.

44. Skoner DP, Rachelefsky GS, Meltzer EO, et al. Detection of growth suppression in children during treatment with intranasal beclomethasone dipropionate. Pediatrics 2000;105(2):E23.

45. Allen DB, Meltzer EO, Lemanske RF, et al. No growth suppression in children treated with the maximum recommended dose of fluticasone propionate aqueous nasal spray for one year. Allergy Asthma Proc 2002;23(6):407–13.

46. Schenkel EJ, Skoner DP, Bronsky EA, et al. Absence of growth retardation in children with perennial allergic rhinitis after one year of treatment with mometasone furoate aqueous nasal spray. Pediatrics 2000;105(2):E22.

47. Brooks CD, Karl KJ, Francom SF. Oral methylprednisolone acetate (Medrol Tablets) for seasonal rhinitis: examination of dose and symptom response. J Clin Pharmacol 1993;33(9):816–22.

48. Snyman JR, Potter PC, Groenewald M, et al, Claricort Study Group. Effect of betamethasone-loratadine combination therapy on severe exacerbations of allergic rhinitis : a randomised, controlled trial. Clin Drug Invest 2004;24(5):265–74.

49. Seidman MD, Gurgel RK, Lin SY, et al. Clinical practice guideline: allergic rhinitis. Otolaryngol Head Neck Surg 2015;152(1 Suppl):S1–43.

50. Sato T, Tareishi Y, Suzuki T, et al. Effect of second-generation antihistamines on nighttime sleep and daytime sleepiness in patients with allergic rhinitis. Sleep Breath 2023. https://doi.org/10.1007/s11325-023-02857-6.

51. Weiner JM, Abramson MJ, Puy RM. Intranasal corticosteroids versus oral H1 receptor antagonists in allergic rhinitis: systematic review of randomised controlled trials. BMJ 1998;317(7173):1624-9.

52. Lieberman P, Kaliner MA, Wheeler WJ. Open-label evaluation of azelastine nasal spray in patients with seasonal allergic rhinitis and nonallergic vasomotor rhinitis. Curr Med Res Opin 2005;21(4):611-8.

53. Nayak AS, Philip G, Lu S, et al. Montelukast fall rhinitis investigator group. efficacy and tolerability of montelukast alone or in combination with loratadine in seasonal allergic rhinitis: a multicenter, randomized, double-blind, placebo-controlled trial performed in the fall. Ann Allergy Asthma Immunol 2002;88(6):592-600.

54. Philip G, Malmstrom K, Hampel FC, et al. Montelukast for treating seasonal allergic rhinitis: a randomized, double-blind, placebo-controlled trial performed in the spring. Clin Exp Allergy 2002;32(7):1020-8.

55. Seresirikachorn K, Mullol J, Limitlaohaphan K, et al. Leukotriene receptor antagonist addition to intranasal steroid: systematic review and meta-analysis. Rhinology 2021;59(1):2-9.

56. Chen ST, Lu KH, Sun HL, et al. Randomized placebo-controlled trial comparing montelukast and cetirizine for treating perennial allergic rhinitis in children aged 2-6 yr. Pediatr Allergy Immunol 2006;17(1):49-54.

57. Clarenbach CF, Kohler M, Senn O, et al. Does nasal decongestion improve obstructive sleep apnea? J Sleep Res 2008;17(4):444-9.

58. Brozek JL, Bousquet J, Baena-Cagnani CE, et al. Allergic rhinitis and its impact on asthma (ARIA) guidelines: 2010 revision. J Allergy Clin Immunol 2010;126(3): 466-76.

59. Cox L, Nelson H, Lockey R, et al. Allergen immunotherapy: a practice parameter third update. J Allergy Clin Immunol 2011;127(1 Suppl):S1-55.

60. Roberts G, Pfaar O, Akdis CA, et al. EAACI guidelines on allergen immunotherapy: allergic rhinoconjunctivitis. Allergy 2018;73(4):765-98.

61. Novakova SM, Staevska MT, Novakova PI, et al. Quality of life improvement after a three-year course of sublingual immunotherapy in patients with house dust mite and grass pollen induced allergic rhinitis: results from real-life. Health Qual Life Outcome 2017;15(1):189.

62. Jacobi H, Rehm D, Nolte H, et al. Effect of house dust mite SLIT-tablet treatment on quality of sleep in allergic rhinitis patients. J Allergy Clin Immunol 2019;143(2): AB286.

63. Kim JY, Jang MJ, Kim DY, et al. Efficacy of subcutaneous and sublingual immunotherapy for house dust mite allergy: a network meta-analysis-based comparison. J Allergy Clin Immunol Pract 2021;9(12):4450-8.e6.

64. Reed J, Talamo M, Tobin MC. Subcutaneous allergen immunotherapy (scit) and its effects on irritability and sleep in patients with allergic rhinitis (ar) utilizing a structured questionnaire. J Allergy Clin Immunol 2015;135(2):AB216.

65. Pitsios C, Tsoumani M, Bilò MB, et al. Contraindications to immunotherapy: a global approach. Clin Transl Allergy 2019;9:45.

66. Chen YL, Tan CT, Huang HM. Long-term efficacy of microdebrider-assisted inferior turbinoplasty with lateralization for hypertrophic inferior turbinates in patients with perennial allergic rhinitis. Laryngoscope 2008;118(7):1270-4.

67. Hamerschmidt R, Hamerschmidt R, Moreira ATR, et al. Comparison of turbinoplasty surgery efficacy in patients with and without allergic rhinitis. Braz J Otorhinolaryngol 2016;82(2):131–9.
68. Parthasarathi K, Christensen JM, Alvarado R, et al. Airflow and symptom outcomes between allergic and non-allergic rhinitis patients from turbinoplasty. Rhinology 2017;55(4):332–8.
69. Anjali PK, Azeem Mohiyuddin SM, Prasad KC, et al. Outcome of submucosal inferior turbinoplasty in perennial allergic rhinitis. Indian J Otolaryngol Head Neck Surg 2022;74(Suppl 2):773–9.
70. Kim SD, Jung DW, Lee JW, et al. Relationship between allergic rhinitis and nasal surgery success in patients with obstructive sleep apnea. Am J Otolaryngol 2021;42(6):103079.
71. Sullivan S, Li K, Guilleminault C. Nasal obstruction in children with sleep-disordered breathing. Ann Acad Med Singapore 2008;37(8):645–8.
72. Zhong J, Luo X, Qiu S, et al. [Preliminary study on efficacy and safety of submucosal plasma ablation of inferior turbinate in children with allergic rhinitis complicated with obstructive sleep apnea syndrome]. Lin Chuang Er Bi Yan Hou Tou Jing Wai Ke Za Zhi 2022;36(10):758–62.

Molecular Allergology and Component-Resolved Diagnosis in Current Clinical Practice

Michael S. Benninger, MD[a],*, Gary A. Falcetano, PA-C[b]

KEYWORDS

- Allergy • Molecular allergology • Component-resolved diagnostics

KEY POINTS

- Specific immunoglobulin E blood testing is a comparable alternative to skin testing to aid in the diagnosis of allergic rhinitis.
- Recent developments in specific component proteins allows for increase fidelity in identifying the true allergens.
- Component resolved diagnostics may become a larger part of the care of individual allergic patients.
- With the ease of allergy blood testing and expanding specific components, the paradigm for allergic management may begin with testing and then identify risk stratification and treatment.

INTRODUCTION

Allergic diseases are highly prevalent conditions and may include a number of clinical manifestations such as allergic rhinitis and sinusitis, dermatologic disorders, conjunctivitis, laryngitis, chronic cough, asthma, and adverse reactions to foods. It is difficult to identify true prevalence rates because diagnosis may not be confirmed, studies may be looking at only one of the allergic diseases and many studies rely on survey responses. When evaluating allergic rhinitis, for example, reported prevalence ranges from 10% to 30% in adults and up to 40% in children.[1,2] Conservative estimates from the Centers for Disease Control suggest in the United States, asthma prevalence has been estimated to be approximately 8.4%, with 7.7% in adults and 9.5% in children.[3]

[a] Department of Otolaryngology-Head and Neck Surgery, Cleveland Clinic Lerner College of Medicine, Head and Neck Institute, The Cleveland Clinic, 9500, Euclid Avenue. A-71, Cleveland, OH 44195, USA; [b] Immuno Diagnostics Division, Thermo Fisher Scientific, 4169 Commercial Avenue, Portage, MI 49002, USA
* Corresponding author.
E-mail address: Benninm@ccf.org

Otolaryngol Clin N Am 57 (2024) 329–342
https://doi.org/10.1016/j.otc.2023.10.003
0030-6665/24/© 2023 Elsevier Inc. All rights reserved.

In the United States alone, the economic burden of asthma-related medical expenses, lost work, and school time and deaths was estimated to be $80 billion yearly.[4]

The diagnosis of allergic disease relies on a classical history based on the patient's perception of specific exposures resulting in symptoms with confirmation by allergy testing or response to treatment. Allergy testing can be performed either through skin tests or in vitro (serologic) testing for specific immunoglobulin E (IgE) directed against potential allergens.[3] In 2015, clinical guidelines for allergic rhinitis were developed by the American Academy of Otolaryngology–Head and Neck Surgery, where it is stated, "Clinicians should perform and interpret, or refer to a clinician who can perform and interpret, specific IgE (skin or blood) allergy testing for patients with a clinical diagnosis of allergic rhinitis (AR) who do not respond to empiric treatment, or when the diagnosis is uncertain, or when knowledge of the specific causative allergen is needed to target therapy."[5]

Allergy testing, whether skin or in vitro testing, can be expensive and is associated with some minor morbidity. Test positivity rates may vary based on the level of suspicion of the ordering provider, the prevalence of specific allergic disease, and the type of clinical practice. Individual allergens can be pursued based on specific symptoms or panels of allergens can be ordered to assess sensitization to a wider range of suspected allergens, these may be additionally grouped by geography. There is also some subjectivity in interpretation of skin test response and the relationship between symptoms and the level of response in skin and IgE testing may be unpredictable.

In an effort to develop a cost-effective allergy test panel, Bousquet and colleagues looked at large numbers of skin allergy tests to identify which tests were highly positive and what size panel might be able to identify the majority of positive allergens. They tested 3034 patients of which 1996 (68.2%) were sensitized to at least one allergen, and identified eight allergens (grass pollen, *Dermatophagoides pteronyssinus*, birch pollen, cat dander, *Artemisia*, olive pollen, *Blatella*, and *Alternaria*) that allowed them to detect more than 95% of sensitized subjects. These studies overlapped a number of European countries which suggested that were some differences observed between countries, but despite these only 13 allergens were needed to identify all sensitized subjects.[6] Although there have been studies evaluating the prevalence of food allergies,[7] there have not been many that have looked at positivity rates of allergy testing for foods.

Our recent studies evaluating large numbers of specific IgE tests showed that "A total of 148,628 results for 48 different allergens were identified. Of the 125,190-potential inhalant/respiratory allergens, the most common positive antigens were dog (24%), cat (23%), dust mites (23% for both D pteronyssinus and Dermatophagoides farina [D farina]) and June grass (21%). Of the 23,438 potential individual food responses, the most common positive allergen tests were milk (18%), peanut (17%), wheat (16%) and egg whites (15%). Most of the results were in Classes 1 to 3, although there were still notable very high Class 5 and Class 6 responses." Therefore, it was found that there was a wide variability of positive in vitro allergy tests, and the likelihood of a positive in allergen panels can be estimated. Evaluating such rates will help to further identify the most and least common allergens and will help to cost-effectively refine allergy assessment panels.[8]

There has been ongoing debate as to whether skin testing or in vitro specific IgE testing are better for patient care, but it is becoming clearer that they are relatively equivalent in relationship to sensitivity and specificity. The 2023 *International Consensus Statement on Allergy and Rhinology: Allergic Rhinitis* (ICAR-AR 2023) document states, "It has been demonstrated that allergen-specific IgE (sIgE) shows excellent correlations with both NPT and SPT in the diagnosis of AR. There is good evidence to show that sIgE is, in many ways, equivalent to SPT."[9] ICAR-AR 2023 also helped to clarify the potential role of specific IgE testing in the management of the allergic patients. "Serum IgE testing offers several benefits. The safety profile of serum IgE testing is the best of all available allergy tests as the risk of anaphylaxis is nonexistent. Furthermore, the use of skin testing is limited in the presence of certain medical conditions. In patients where skin testing is contraindicated or potentially impacted by medications, sIgE [allergen-specific IgE] testing offers a safe and effective option for determining the presence of sensitization as a biomarker of IgE-mediated hypersensitivity and confirming specific allergen triggers."[9]

One of the major issues with skin or specific IgE testing is that the test may recognize an immune reaction to a specific protein, but that protein may be present in more than one allergen and the testing may be identifying a cross-reactivity rather than the original sensitization. Therefore, the treatment strategies avoidance or allergen immunotherapy may not truly select for the preferred targeted allergen. Recent developments and refinements of serum IgE testing allows for a more individualized approach to identifying specific allergens by evaluating the discrete allergen components, mostly proteins, unique to each allergen. This evaluation is referred to as component-resolved diagnostics (CRD) or allergen component testing. This article discusses the use of CRD in the evaluation and treatment of allergic disease.

THE BASICS OF COMPONENT-RESOLVED DIAGNOSTICS

An allergen contains thousands of molecules but only a few of these molecules are allergenic to humans. Each allergen has a number of components, which are generally proteins, and each of these allergens has different characteristics, which may impact the effects of sensitization. Species-specific components are typically unique to the allergen and can be evaluated to determine if the component sensitization is also specific. Because many of these proteins can be found in multiple allergens, it is the specificity of the unique component(s) that helps to determine if a person is truly sensitized to that allergen. Furthermore, each of these components has specific characteristics, which impact the effects of sensitization. Sensitization to cross-reactive components may suggest that the sensitivity noted in traditional whole extract-based allergy testing may be from one of these cross-reacting components and not to the specific proteins of those allergens. The ability to identify components that are unique to an allergen or that may be cross-reactive to other allergens helps to identify the true sources of sensitization.

In 1991, it was first shown that recombinant allergens could be used for the in vitro diagnosis of allergy.[10] The first studies used immunoblot to make this assessment. The mRNA is isolated from a particular allergen source. This is then cloned, and a specific DNA sequence is produced. The sequence is then identified for its specific allergen structure and used in the diagnosis of the specific allergen that causes sensitization.[11] Each of the allergen components can be evaluated to determine if the patient is sensitized to the allergen-specific protein or one of the cross-reacting components.

Component analysis allows for the determination of sensitization to the allergen-specific component or cross-reacting component and thereby allows for the assessment of the true sensitization. Because skin testing and specific IgE testing may be positive due to the cross-reacting proteins, a positive test may not determine true symptomatic sensitization. In addition, specific components may induce different clinical responses, depending on certain characteristics which can affect the consequences of sensitization. Although this article could identify hundreds of ways that specific component assessment can be used for the refinement of allergy diagnosis, the authors highlight three in particular, food allergy (particularly peanut and tree nut), pet allergy, and an example of the use of component analysis to identify symptomatic sensitivity in cross-reacting allergens from different unique pollen sources.

Food Allergy: Component-Resolved Diagnosis

Food allergy is very common, especially in the pediatric population. The most common food allergies are milk, peanut, tree nut, wheat, egg white, soybean, fish, shellfish, and sesame.[8,12] Because certain components such as profilins and cross-reactive carbohydrate determinants (CCDs) are ubiquitous in nature, it is often difficult with standard allergy testing to be sure that the clinical symptoms are due to the allergen identified on skin or sIgE test results. Component testing can be useful in such circumstance to identify the true sensitization.

Probably, the most dramatic of the specific component characteristics is in foods where stability or lability of foods once they are processed in the gut will impact the clinical symptoms. Stability of allergens depends on several factors, including the molecular weight of the proteins, hydrophilicity, and the contact surface. Allergens that enter through the respiratory tract can be low molecular weight and can have low stability. Allergens have more difficulty crossing the skin barrier. Those that enter via the digestive tract, such as foods are exposed to proteases and food processing, so they must have high stability to avoid breakdown.[13] Disulfide bonds contribute to protein stability and help to create a three-dimensional structure where IgE binding is preserved, resulting in resistance to proteolytic enzyme degradation.[13] Egg is particularly sensitive to degradation not only in the gastrointestinal (GI) tract but with cooking, so that many egg allergic patients do not have a clinical reaction to extensively heated eggs. Assessing for the presence of allergen component proteins that are resistant to heat degradation such as ovomucoid in the egg and casein in milk can aid in the diagnosis of those patients who will not tolerate egg and milk in any form including extensively heated foods like muffins and cakes.

Peanut and Tree Nuts

The diagnosis of peanut and tree nut allergy can range from straightforward to complex. As with any allergy diagnosis, the history, physical examination, and prevalence in the population must guide the selection and interpretation of diagnostic testing.

Whole extract testing for peanut- and tree nut-specific IgE by either skin prick test (SPT) or in vitro serologic assay is routinely used as the primary method of assessing relevant IgE antibody response. Correlated with a clear history of a systemic reaction, this may be all that is necessary to confirm a clinical allergy to peanut or tree nuts.[11]

However, sometimes, the history is unclear, and additional diagnostics may be helpful in reaching an ultimate diagnosis. The availability of single molecular peanut and tree nut allergen components has added additional diagnostic specificity and often provides a basis to predict, on a more individual level, a patient's potential clinical response to ingestion of the suspected food.[11,13] Understanding the properties of these individual components can inform clinical management and further diagnostic procedures such as whether an oral food challenge (OFC) should be performed.[11] When used appropriately, component-resolved peanut diagnostics can help clinicians to evaluate the risks involved, potentially increasing the number of low-risk OFCs, and when appropriate eventually leading to "de-labeling" of an allergy diagnosis. Alternatively, the components can also indicate when a high-risk situation exists, potentially reducing the number of failed OFCs performed.[11] For clinicians that do not perform

OFCs themselves, this information can inform appropriate referrals to those specialists that do.

As detailed in **Fig. 1**, peanut and tree nut allergen component families can be considered on a stratified "risk ramp" with heat and digestion stable proteins being associated with the greatest risk of systemic reactions.[11]

Seed Storage Proteins

Allergen components demonstrating the highest risk of clinical reactions are the seed storage proteins.[13] Tree nuts and legumes such as peanut contain storage proteins such as 2S albumins and 7S and 11S globulins, these are predominantly "species specific" and demonstrate the least cross-reactivity with proteins found in other plant foods and pollens. Storage proteins are highly abundant in plant foods and are resistant to denaturing by both heat and digestive enzymes.[11] Examples of storage proteins associated with the highest risk of clinical reactions are the members of the 2S albumin family; Ara h 2 and Ara h 6 in the peanut, Ana o 3 in cashew, Cor a 14 in hazelnut, Ber e 1 in brazil nut, Jug r 1 in walnut, and Ses i 1 in sesame seed. These 2S albumins have all been identified as significantly predictive of clinical reactions to their related foods.[13]

Nonspecific Lipid Transfer Proteins

Non-specific lipid transfer proteins also known as lipid transfer proteins (LTPs) present some unique challenges from a clinical standpoint when attempting to evaluate their ability to cause systemic symptoms in sensitized patients. They are typically considered to be of variable risk. Patients sensitized to LTPs, such as Ara h 9 in peanut and Cor a 8 in hazelnut, may exhibit symptoms ranging from pollen food (oral allergy) syndrome to anaphylaxis. Like storage proteins, they are highly abundant in plant foods and are resistant to denaturing by both heat and digestive enzymes.[11] Unlike storage proteins, however, their location is not restricted to seed tissues, but ubiquitously expressed throughout the plant.[11] LTPs mostly exhibit a high degree of cross-reactivity with homologous LTPs in other plant foods and pollens. This cross-reactivity with pollens is thought to promote the sensitization and subsequent development of associated plant food allergy.[11] Geographic location seems to play a unique role in allergic responses for patients sensitized to LTPs. Populations in

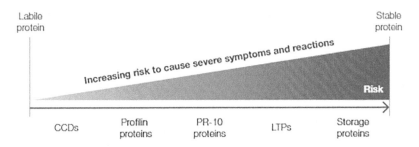

An overview of the biological differences in how allergen proteins can cause different types of symptoms

Fig. 1. Individual allergen component proteins and their association to the risk of clinical symptoms. (Reproduced with permission from Thermo Fisher Scientific.)

Mediterranean countries seem to represent the highest prevalence of LTP-related clinical food allergy.[11]

Pathogenesis Related-10 Proteins

The remaining allergen components have decreasing levels of clinical significance from Ara h 8 in the peanut and Cor a 1 in hazelnuts, which are pathogenesis related-10 (PR-10) proteins that are homologous to Fagales family of pollens (eg, birch). Ara h 8 and Cor a 1 are labile and can be denatured by digestive enzymes making systemic symptoms from sensitization to them unlikely. Those individuals that do exhibit symptoms related to PR-10 proteins have symptoms that are typically confined to the oropharynx, and this is commonly referred to as "pollen food allergy syndrome" or "oral allergy syndrome." The PR-10 family of proteins is very cross-reactive. This cross-reactivity often accounts for clinically insignificant whole allergen extract positive assays of PR-10 containing plant foods such as peanuts and tree nuts in patients that are sensitized to pollen proteins such as birch Bet v 1, a homologous protein to Ara h 8 and Cor a 1 in peanuts and hazelnuts, respectively.[14,15]

Cross-Reactive Carbohydrate Determinates and Profilins

Other peanut and tree nut allergen components that are highly cross-reactive with pollens and typically are not associated with symptoms of clinical allergy, include profilins and CCDs. Profilins and CCDs are ubiquitous in nature and are present in all plants and pollens. Both CCDs and profilins are labile molecules that are denatured by digestive enzymes.[11,14]

The structures of profilins are highly conserved within different species. This allows the assessment of sensitizations to be accomplished by assaying a single representative allergen such as Bet v 2 in birch pollen or Phl p 12 in timothy grass pollen as surrogates for the entire profilin family. Similarly, assessing for a single cross-reactive carbohydrate marker such as MUXF3 allows for a thorough assessment of CCD sensitizations from pollens and plant food sources.[11]

Fig. 2 displays the most commonly used and commercially available peanut and tree nut, soy, sesame, and wheat allergen components in the risk ramp format.

Risk stratification

	CCD	Profilin	PR-10	LTP	Storage Protein
Peanut	MUXF3	Bet v 2*	Ara h 8	Ara h 9	Ara h 1, 2, 3, 6
Hazelnut	MUFX3	Bet v 2*	Cor a 1	Cor a 8	Cor a 9, 14
Walnut	MUFX3	Bet v 2*		Jug r 3	Jug r 1
Brazil nut	MUFX3	Bet v 2*			Ber e 1
Cashew	MUFX3	Bet v 2*			Ana o 3
Wheat	MUXF3	Phl p 12*		Tri a 14	Gliadin† (α-, β-, γ- and ω-gliadin) Tri a 19 (ω-5-gliadin)
Sesame					Ses i 1
Soy	MUXF3	Bet v 2*	Gly m 4		Gly m 5, 6

Fig. 2. Risk and cross-reactivity ramp illustrating commonly available allergen components. (Reproduced with permission from Thermo Fisher Scientific.)

SESAME AND WHEAT ALLERGEN COMPONENTS

Recently available in the United States, sesame and wheat allergen components improve the diagnostic specificity and in the case of wheat, sensitivity as well, for these two increasingly prevalent food allergies that have thus far proven challenging to diagnose.

Sesame Allergy

Sesame allergen component Ses i 1 is a seed storage protein and member of the 2S albumin family. As is the case with the other 2S albumins like Ara h 2 and 6 in the peanut, Ses i 1 adds to the specificity of sesame allergy diagnosis with elevated levels not only indicative of true sesame allergy but also being predictive of increased severity of reactions.[16–23]

Wheat Allergy

In the case of suspected wheat allergy, the newly available wheat components add a level of improved diagnosis in what has previously been a challenging diagnostic dilemma. Whole extract wheat assays and skin testing extracts can demonstrate irrelevant positive results due to cross-reactivity with ubiquitous plant pollens that a patient may be sensitized to. Wheat, being a grain in the grass family, commonly demonstrates this cross-reactive phenomenon in grass allergic patients. In addition, the whole allergen wheat extracts can a lack full representation of gliadins, including the omega-5 gliadin Tri a 19, due to differences in solubility of the individual proteins. This underrepresentation of the gliadins necessitates the initial testing of both whole extract wheat and gliadins upfront before subsequent reflex testing of Tri a 19 from the gliadins and Tri a 14 along with CCD and profilin, from the whole extract wheat (see **Fig. 3**).

The newly available wheat allergen components such as gliadin (Tri a 19) and Tri a 14 add to the specificity of wheat allergy diagnosis. All three have been correlated with clinical wheat allergy as opposed to clinically irrelevant sensitization. In addition, Tri a 19 (omega-5 gliadin) plays an important role in the uncommon but unique syndrome of wheat-dependent exercise-induced anaphylaxis (WDEIA). This condition is manifested by clinical symptoms to wheat ingestion occurring only in association with strenuous exercise with symptoms appearing sometimes hours after the ingestion of wheat-containing foods. Tri a 19 (omega-5 gliadin) is the main allergen component of wheat that is associated with this syndrome. The other gliadins (alpha, beta,

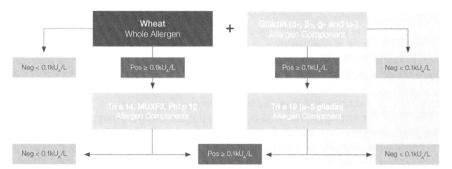

Fig. 3. Diagnostic pathway for suspected wheat allergy. (Reproduced with permission from Thermo Fisher Scientific.)

gamma) and Tri a 14 have also been identified as predictive of WDEIA but to a lesser extent than Tri a 19.

Tri a 14 is a nonselective lipid transfer protein which is not only associated with clinical wheat allergy and WDEIA but also a condition known as Baker's allergy (or Baker's asthma). This condition is a respiratory allergy, usually occupational in nature, which develops mainly in bakers or others with high exposure to airborne wheat allergens. Finally, the highly ubiquitous but usually benign cross-reactive pan-allergen components that are present in plant pollens and also in wheat, CCDs, and profilins mentioned earlier also play a role here in identifying the drivers of clinically irrelevant wheat sensitization.[24–30]

ALPHA-GAL SYNDROME: DELAYED MAMMALIAN (RED) MEAT ALLERGY

This very unique allergic condition, identified only within the past 20 years or so, is an allergy that develops after one, or more commonly, several bites of a tick, which sensitizes the host to the glycan galactose-alpha-1,3-galactose (alpha-Gal), an oligosaccharide that is present in all mammals with the exception of humans and old world primates. The lone star tick (*Amblyomma americanum*) in North America is considered the main vector of sensitization; however, it is suspected that other insect vectors such as chiggers or seed ticks may be involved as well.

It is not just the mode of sensitization that is unique but also the agenesis. Unlike traditional type I hypersensitivity reactions, alpha-gal-related symptoms can present in a delayed manner sometimes as long as 8 hours after an ingestion or exposure. Severe reactions including anaphylaxis are common, but more moderate symptoms are also encountered including isolated gastrointestinal distress and urticaria. These moderate symptoms can be chronic in nature especially in patients with a consistent diet of mammalian meats. SPT in vivo testing is not recommended as results are often falsely negative. Serologic testing for alpha-gal-specific IgE allergen components is the diagnostic test of choice and is widely available from laboratories.[31–33]

FURRY ANIMALS

Pet allergies, particularly dogs and cats, are among the most common allergies. Many patients who test positive for dog also test positive for cat, and they can also test positive for horse. Although patients may be truly sensitized to all three of these, at times it is the cross-sensitization of nonspecific components that do not cause symptoms but result in the positive testing. The primary allergenic lipocalins are Can f 1 and Can f 2 for dog, Fel d 1 and Fel d 4 for cat, and Equ c 1 for horse. The use of specific component testing can be used to define the true sensitization. **Fig. 4** illustrates the currently identified pet allergen components for horses, dogs, and cats, respectively.

In the case of a symptomatic patient where the true animal sensitivity is not clear and where there is a positive skin or in vitro sIgE test, component analysis can be used to clarify which animals the patient is truly allergic to. The example below in **Fig. 5** shows a suspected allergy to dog with positive testing also to horse and cat. By identifying the animal-specific components and going through an elimination process, the true sensitizing allergy can be identified.

One of the interesting phenomena in pet dog dander allergy is that up to 40% of dog allergic patients are monosensitized to the prostate protein Can f 5, and if this is identified as the only protein, the patient could tolerate a female dog or a dog that was neutered before maturation. Furthermore, a clinical benefit of assessing pet allergen components is the ability to better predict both the development of future disease and the severity of disease as well. In a population-based longitudinal study from

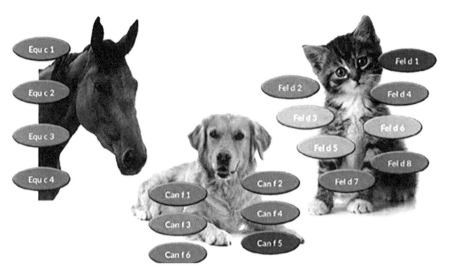

Fig. 4. Known components for horse, dog, and cat. (*From* Matricardi PM, Klein-Tebbe J, Hoffman HJ, Valenta R, Ollert M, Eds. EAACI Molecular Allergology: User's Guide. Pediatr Allergy Immunol, 2016; 27(Suppl23):1–250.)

Sweden, Asarnoj and colleagues demonstrated that the more individual cat or dog allergen components a child was sensitized to at age 4 year the greater the likelihood of developing clinical disease by age 16 year.[34] Additional researchers, such as Patelis and Konradsen and colleagues, have demonstrated a similar relationship with an increasing number of furry animal component allergen sensitizations being correlated with increasing severity of disease.[35,36] This additional information allows clinicians to base their management recommendations on the risks involved in continued animal exposure and may determine how prescriptive advice such as pet avoidance or immunotherapy should be.

With sophisticated analysis, the true sensitizations related to furry animals can be assessed. Such an algorithm can also be set up for any allergen grouping such as trees, grasses, or weeds.

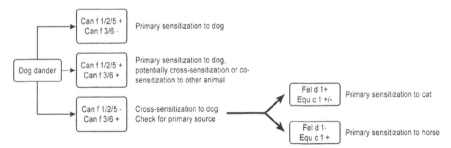

Fig. 5. The value of the use of specific component analysis in a patient with a positive IgE test for dog dander. (*From* Matricardi PM, Klein-Tebbe J, Hoffman HJ, Valenta R, Ollert M, Eds. EAACI Molecular Allergology: User's Guide. Pediatr Allergy Immunol, 2016; 27(Suppl23):1–250.)

USING COMPONENT ANALYSIS TO IDENTIFY ALLERGY IN CROSS-REACTIVITY AMONG TYPES OF ALLERGENS

One of the problems in identifying the true sensitization in individuals who are polysensitized is that many components within an allergen are common across other allergens. This is particularly true for the profilin, polcalcin, and CCDs. A very good example illustrated in **Fig. 6** is mugwort, birch, and timothy. The allergens come from three different allergen groups, weeds, tree, and grass. A skin or in vitro sIgE test may be positive to all of them due to the shared profilin and polcalcin found in all of them. Specific components for timothy include Phl p 1 and Phl p 5. If these are positive but species-specific components to mugwort and birch are not identified, then the true sensitivity is to timothy grass.

USING COMPONENT TESTING TO REFINE ALLERGY ASSESSMENT

Component testing can be valuable in determining the true sensitizing allergen, refining specific treatment and determining the best antigens for immunotherapy. The use of component testing is probably less valuable in monosensitized patients but can be invaluable in polysensitized individuals. The more positive tests that there are by skin or sIgE testing the more likely that some of these may be due to cross-sensitization. Therefore, as depicted in **Fig. 7**, the utility of molecular component testing becomes more valuable in the management of their allergic disease. It is also more valuable where the risks of exposure on clinical symptoms are high such as in peanut allergy, where the risk of anaphylaxis can be assessed.[14]

This approach to testing can also be used where the abundance of molecules in whole extract is low or when the stability of a single allergen is low. In such cases, molecular assessment can be especially useful. Molecular testing can also be adopted to transform an allergy practice. If an individual has symptomatic allergy, skin tests or in vitro sIgE testing can be obtained. If they are monosensitized or there are few positive tests and the individual is symptomatic to these allergens, then avoidance, pharmacotherapy, or immunotherapy can be initiated. If, however, the individual is

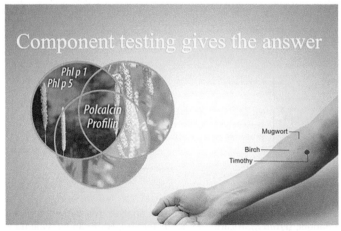

Fig. 6. Positive test to Phl p 1 and Phl p 5 identify the sensitizing allergen as timothy. (Reproduced with permission from Thermo Fisher Scientific.)

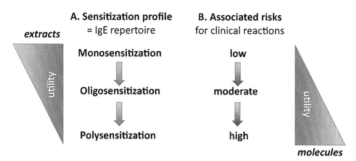

Fig. 7. Utility of molecular testing in patients who are polysensitized or those with risk for high clinical reactions. (*From* Matricardi PM, Klein-Tebbe J, Hoffman HJ, Valenta R, Ollert M, Eds. EAACI Molecular Allergology: User's Guide. Pediatr Allergy Immunol, 2016; 27(Suppl23):1–250.)

polysensitized or sensitized to allergens that impart a high clinical risk, then molecular component testing can be performed to identify the true allergens and initiate treatment accordingly.

Another potential option is to use IgE blood testing (and also likely component testing) to create phenotypes which could help aid in refining treatment, reduce morbidity, and reduce cost. A phenotype for potentially poorly manageable allergic asthmatics has been identified, using emergency room visits, hospitalizations, and systemic steroid rescues as measures of difficult to control asthma. Patients with higher class of IgE response (3+ or greater) and allergies to dog, cat, house dust, and some molds were associated with more severe asthma. With better association of specific IgE and component-resolved diagnostics, specific phenotypes and paradigms for evaluation and treatment will be able to be accomplished.[37]

As component testing becomes easier to perform using large numbers of components and becomes less expensive, then it is foreseeable that component testing at the outset, and then working backwards to whether or not the patient is symptomatic to the identified allergens. In some cases, it can even be used to identify at risk patients before significant symptomatology. An example of this is that children who test positive to Bet v 1 (birch) at an early age are more likely to have more significant respiratory symptoms by age 16 year.[15] With the development of microarray chips where multiple components can be assessed with only a few drops of blood, the ability to identify allergic disease simply and efficiently has become a reality.[38]

SUMMARY

Allergy diagnosis continues to evolve as molecular diagnostics are developed, refined, and adopted into regular clinical practice. Whole allergen extracts remain the current first-line diagnostic choice due to their superior sensitivity, CRD, where available, generally improve on specificity allowing for a more precise diagnosis and consequently a more personalized management plan. Although, as we have seen with wheat, CRD can also improve on sensitivity for allergen extracts that may underrepresent important allergen component proteins. Understanding the benefits and limitations of the currently available diagnostics along with importance of correlating any testing with the patients' medical history will allow clinicians to provide the best possible care to their patients with suspected IgE-mediated disease.

CLINICS CARE POINTS

- Selection of allergy diagnostic testing should always be guided by a thorough history.
- Interpretation of allergy diagnostic testing should take into account pretest probability based on patient history and prevalence in the population.
- Molecular characterization of allergic sensitizations can provide information that allows for a more precise understanding of the clinical implications for an individual patient, facilitating a more personalized diagnosis and management plan.

DISCLOSURE

M Benninger is a consultant for Thermo-Fisher and research funding from Merck, United States and APMed. G Falcetano is an employee of Thermo-Fisher Diagnostics.

REFERENCES

1. McCrory DC, Williams JW, Dolor RJ, et al. Management of allergic rhinitis in the working-age population. Evid Rep Technol Assess 2003;67:1–4.
2. Andersson M. Emerging treatments for allergic rhinitis. Expert Opin Emerg Drugs 2003;8:63–9.
3. Centers for Disease Control and Prevention. Asthma facts—CDC's national asthma control program grantees. Atlanta, GA: U.S. Department of Health and Human Services, Centers for Disease Control and Prevention; 2013.
4. Nurmagambetov T, Kuwahara R, Garbe P. The Economic Burden of Asthma in the United States, 2008-2013. Ann Am Thorac Soc 2018;15(3):348–56.
5. Seidman MD, Gurgel RK, Lin SY, et al, Guideline Otolaryngology Development Group. AAO-HNSF. Clinical practice guideline: allergic rhinitis. Otolaryngol Head Neck Surg 2015;152(1S):S1–4.
6. Bousquet PJ, Burbach G, Heinzerling LM, et al. GA2LEN skin test study III: Minimum battery of test inhalent allergens needed in epidemiological studies in patients. Allergy 2009;64:1656–62.
7. Sampson HA. Update on food allergy. J Allergy Clin Immunol 2004;113: 805–8019.
8. Benninger MS, Grafmiller K, Yong V, et al. Relationship between specific atopic diseases and in-vitro allergic sensitivities. Ear Nose Throat J 2018;97:296–322.
9. Wise SK, Lin SY, Toskala E, et al. International consensus statement on allergy and rhinology: Allergic rhinitis. Int Forum Allergy Rhinol 2018;8:108–352.
10. Valenta R, Duchene M, Vrtala S, et al. Receombinant allergens for immunoblot diagnosis of tree-pollen allergy. J Allergy Clin Immunol 1991;88:889–94.
11. EAACI Molecular Allergology: User's Guide. In: Matricardi PM, Klein-Tebbe J, Hoffman HJ, et al, editors. Pediatr Allergy Immunol 2016;27(Suppl23):1–250.
12. https://www.fda.gov/food/food-labeling-nutrition/food-allergies.
13. Pekar J Ret D, Untersmayr E, Untersmayr E. Stability of allergens. Mol Immunol 2018;100:14–20.
14. Steering Committee Authors; Review Panel Members. A WAO - ARIA - GA2LEN consensus document on molecular-based allergy diagnosis (PAMD@): Update 2020. World Allergy Organ J 2020;13(2):100091.
15. Westman M, Lupinek C, Bousquet J, et al. Early childhood IgE reactivity to pathogenesis-related class 10 proteins predicts allergic rhinitis in adolescence. J Allergy Clin Immunol 2014;135:1199–206.

16. Borres M, Maruyama N, Sato S, et al. Recent advances in component resolved diagnosis in food allergy. Allergol Int 2016;65(4):378–87.

17. Sato S, Yanagida N, Ebisawa M. How to diagnose food allergy. Curr Opin Allergy Clin Immunol 2018;18(3):214–21.

18. Foong RX, Dantzer JA, Wood RA, et al. Improving diagnostic accuracy in food allergy. J Allergy Clin Immunol Pract 2021;9(1):71–80.

19. Maruyama N, Nakagawa T, Ito K, et al. Measurement of specific IgE antibodies to Ses i 1 improves the diagnosis of sesame allergy. Clin Exp Allergy 2016;46(1): 163–71.

20. Yanagida N, Ejiri Y, Takeishi D, et al. Ses i 1-specific IgE and sesame oral food challenge results. J Allergy Clin Immunol Pract 2019;7(6):2084–6.

21. Saf S, Sifers TM, Baker MG, et al. Diagnosis of Sesame Allergy: Analysis of Current Practice and Exploration of Sesame Component Ses i 1. J Allergy Clin Immunol Pract 2020;8(5):1681–8.

22. Goldberg MR, Appel MY, Nachshon L, et al. Combinatorial advantage of Ses i 1-specific IgE and Basophil Activation for diagnosis of Sesame Food Allergy. Pediatr Allergy Immunol 2021. https://doi.org/10.1111/pai.13533. Online ahead of print.

23. Nachshon L, Goldberg MR, Levy MB, et al. Efficacy and Safety of Sesame Oral Immunotherapy – A Real-World, Single-Center Study. J Allergy Clin Immunol Pract 2019;7:2775–81.

24. Ito K, Futamura M, Borres MP, et al. IgE antibodies to omega-5 gliadin associate with immediate symptoms on oral wheat challenge in Japanese children. Allergy 2008;63(11):1536–42.

25. Cianferoni A. Wheat allergy: diagnosis and management. J Asthma Allergy 2016; 9:13–25.

26. Palacin A, Varela J, Quirce S, et al. Recombinant lipid transfer protein Tri a 14: a novel heat and proteolytic resistant tool for the diagnosis of baker's asthma. Clin Exp Allergy 2009;39(8):1267–76.

27. Kotaniemi-Syrjänen A, Palosuo K, Jartti T, et al. The prognosis of wheat hypersensitivity in children. Pediatr Allergy Immunol 2010;21(2 Pt 2):e421–8.

28. Sandiford CP, Tatham AS, Fido R, et al. Identification of the major water/salt insoluble wheat proteins involved in cereal hypersensitivity. Clin Exp Allergy 1997; 27(10):1120–9.

29. Nilsson N, Sjölander S, Baar A, et al. Wheat allergy in children evaluated with challenge and IgE antibodies to wheat components. Pediatr Allergy Immunol 2015;26(2):119–25.

30. Hofmann SC, Fischer J, Eriksson C, et al. IgE detection to α/β/γ-gliadin and its clinical relevance in wheat-dependent exercise-induced anaphylaxis. Allergy 2012;67(11):1457–60.

31. Commins SP, Satinover SM, Hosen J, et al. Delayed anaphylaxis, angioedema, or urticaria after consumption of red meat in patients with IgE antibodies specific for galactose-alpha-1,3-galactose. J Allergy Clin Immunol 2009;123(2):426–33.

32. Commins SP, Platts-Mills TA. Allergenicity of carbohydrates and their role in anaphylactic events. Curr Allergy Asthma Rep 2010;10(1):29–33.

33. Steinke JW, Platts-Mills TA, Commins SP. The alpha-gal story: lessons learned from connecting the dots. J Allergy Clin Immunol 2015;135(3):589–96, quiz 597.

34. Asarnoj A, Hamsten C, Wadén K, et al. Sensitization to cat and dog allergen molecules in childhood and prediction of symptoms of cat and dog allergy in adolescence: A BAMSE/MeDALL study. J Allergy Clin Immunol 2016;137(3):813–21.e7.

35. Patelis A, Gunnbjornsdottir M, Alving K, et al. Allergen extract vs. component sensitization and airway inflammation, responsiveness and new-onset respiratory disease. Clin Exp Allergy 2016;46(5):730–40.

36. Konradsen JR, Nordlund B, Onell A, et al. Severe childhood asthma and allergy to furry animals: refined assessment using molecular-based allergy diagnostics. Pediatr Allergy Immunol 2014;25(2):187–92.

37. Benninger MS, Caberar CI, Amador EM, et al. Phenotypes of allergic asthma: Does in-vitro allergy testing help to predict asthma severity? Am J Rhino Allergy 2022;36(6):755–62.

38. Lupinek C, Wollman F, Baar A, et al. Advances in allergen-microarray technology for diagnosis and monitoring of allergy: The MeDALL allergen chip. Methods 2014;106:106–19.

Eosinophilic Esophagitis
What the Otolaryngologist Needs to Know

Nainika Nanda, MD, Dinesh Chhetri, MD*

KEYWORDS

- Eosinophilic esophagitis • Dysphagia • Food impaction • GERD • Atopy • Allergen
- Biologic

KEY POINTS

- Eosinophilic esophagitis is a male-predominant disorder in adults and children.
- Pathophysiology includes (1) immunoglobulin E (IgE) and non-IgE–mediated allergic responses and (2) epithelial barrier impairment.
- Symptoms include the following:
  - Pediatrics: feeding intolerance, nausea and vomiting, and failure to thrive.
  - Adults: dysphagia and food impaction, heartburn, and chest pain.
- Diagnosis relies on acquiring adequate history, endoscopic findings, and multiple mucosal biopsies.
- Treatment is based on 3 paradigms:
  - Diet: elemental diets and elimination diets.
  - Drugs: topical corticosteroid, proton-pump inhibitor, dupilumab.
  - Dilation is reserved for symptomatic and anatomic management because it does not alter the underlying pathologic inflammation.

EPIDEMIOLOGY

Eosinophilic esophagitis (EOE) was first recognized in the 1990s. Since its designation as a distinct clinical entity, increased understanding of the pathophysiology and management of the disease has emerged. The prevalence of EOE in the United States is estimated to be from 30.9 to 71.9 per 100,000 cases. Previous reports have suggested prevalence varying based on region (highest to lowest: Midwest states, northeastern states, west states).[1] Additionally, male prevalence is higher, making up around 75% of cases.[1]

Department of Head & Neck Surgery, University of California Los Angeles, 200 UCLA Medical Plaza, Suite 550, Los Angeles, CA 90024, USA
* Corresponding author.
E-mail address: dchhetri@mednet.ucla.edu

Otolaryngol Clin N Am 57 (2024) 343–352
https://doi.org/10.1016/j.otc.2023.10.004
0030-6665/24/© 2023 Elsevier Inc. All rights reserved.

PATHOPHYSIOLOGY

Pathophysiology of the disease has been debated. A genetic component is believed to exist because male first-degree relatives have an increased risk of disease development. Genes involved in atopic disease have been implicated, such as thymic stromal lymphopoietin, which regulates Th2 cell development and eosinophilic activation. Additionally, more specific genes and epigenetic regulation have been implicated as well, such as eosinophil chemoattractant, chemokine ligand 26 (CCL26), and esophageal epithelial barrier gene, CAPN14.[2–5] However, the inheritance is complex and may be overestimated, based on twin studies that account for common environment.[6]

Therefore, genetics alone cannot account for disease phenotype. Given the similarities of EOE and other atopic diseases along with the up to 70% presence of concomitant atopic disease in affected individuals, the role of allergens has been investigated.[7–9] The majority of affected patients have positive skin prick and atopy patch tests, prompting the theory of immunoglobulin E (IgE) and non-IgE–mediated allergic responses in disease manifestation.[10,11] This response is driven by allergens reacting with IgE bound to mast cells, leading to mast cell degranulation. Degranulation results in the release of histamine and chemotactic factors, such as interleukin (IL)-5, that recruit eosinophils. Through a Th2 response, IL-5 drives eosinophil maturation and migration. These eosinophils then release a variety of factors that drive inflammation. In fact, IgE-bearing mast cells have even been found in esophageal tissue of patients without atopy or positive allergy testing.[12] Further support of this allergen response theory is demonstrated in murine models, where challenge with aeroallergens and ovalbumin or overexpression of human EOE cytokines can sensitize and induce EOE phenotype.[13–15] Specifically, IL-5 has been implicated. IL-5 null murine models develop less eosinophilia in esophageal tissue exposed to allergens as compared with wild type mice. Conversely, treatment with anti-IL-5 antibodies can decrease the number of esophageal eosinophils.[16,17]

Pathogenesis of EOE has also been attributed to epithelial barrier impairment, demonstrated by dilated interepithelial spaces, altered epithelial barrier function, and downregulation of barrier function proteins and adhesion molecules.[18–20] This altered epithelial barrier can lead to increased permeability that enhances antigen presentation, resulting in recruitment of eosinophils.

SYMPTOMS

Disease presentation varies with age. Younger patients often have nonspecific complaints, such as feeding intolerance, nausea and vomiting, and failure to thrive.[8] With age, dysphagia and food impaction become more common. Additionally, heartburn and chest pain can be presenting symptoms.[21] Symptoms are often more severe with dense, dry, rough-textured foods, such as bread and meats. With ongoing symptoms, adaptive behaviors can develop, such as eating slowly, prolonged mastication, increased fluid intake with food, crushing pills, or taking small bites, which can make parsing out the characteristics of dysphagia increasingly challenging.

Several scoring systems have been proposed but are not well validated, uniformly accepted, or promoted by EOE clinical guidelines. One simplified score, the Dysphagia Symptom Questionnaire, a 3-question patient-reported outcome, is administered during 30 days and has excellent compliance and acceptance. However, it is critiqued by its limited focus on dysphagia.[22] Another proposed instrument, Eosinophilic Esophagitis Activity Index PRO, is validated for adult patients. This 7-item questionnaire asks patients to recall dysphagia symptoms during a 7-day period, considering adaptive behaviors.[23] However, this also has limited accuracy (60%–65%) when compared to endoscopic and histologic findings.[24]

DIAGNOSIS

Diagnostic criteria consist of symptoms of esophageal dysfunction, tissue biopsy via endoscopy, and exclusion of other non-EOE disorders that can increase esophageal eosinophilia.

Examination via endoscopy can demonstrate trachealization (fixed esophageal rings), longitudinal furrows, white exudates, mucosal pallor or edema, narrowing of esophageal caliber, "crepe paper esophagus" (friable mucosa), and strictures.[25] Because these findings are nonspecific to EOE, biopsy is required.

Biopsy review can be challenging. Highly specific histologic features of eosinophilia, often found layered within the epithelium, include lamina propria fibrosis and eosinophils aggregated in microabscesses. However, these features are rarely present.[22] The eosinophilic infiltrate can also extend to deeper layers via disrupted epithelial tight junctions, resulting in eventual collagen deposition and macroscopic tissue remodeling. Samples obtained should include a minimum of 2 to 4 biopsies from the distal esophagus and 2 to 4 from the proximal esophagus, with a minimum of 6 biopsies from grossly inflamed tissue.[9] A diagnostic biopsy contains esophageal eosinophilia of 15 eosinophils/high powered field ($\sim$60 eos/mm^2) or greater. Diagnostic sensitivities based on this cutoff in one study were 84%, 97%, and 100% when obtaining 2, 3, and 6 biopsy specimens, respectively.[26] However, a positive biopsy by eosinophil count alone is not pathognomonic for EOE. Other disorders that can result in positive biopsy for esophageal eosinophilia include hypereosinophilic syndrome, eosinophilic gastroenteritis, infection, vasculitis, celiac disease, and Crohn disease. Therefore, history, examination, and biopsy are required for diagnosis.

Additionally, the most recent update to consensus guidelines for EOE in 2018 has recognized that gastroesophageal reflux disease (GERD) can be concurrently present.[27] Whereas in the past, proton pump inhibitor (PPI) responsiveness was used to differentiate GERD from EOE. GERD is theorized to cause acid-induced mucosal injury. This generates an inflammatory response, which induces mucosal eosinophilic infiltration and antigen exposure. Conversely, the presence of EOE can increase the risk of GERD via altered mucosal barrier function.[28]

Barium esophagram can be used to identify anatomic abnormalities from tissue remodeling, such as stenosis and strictures. Novel diagnostic modalities have been developed to combat the cost burden and risk of mucosal disruption with endoscopy, although these modalities have not been shown to offer clear benefit.[29] These include mucosal impedance testing, impedance planimetry, esophageal string, cytosponge, allergy and esophageal prick testing, high-resolution esophageal manometry, endoscopic ultrasonography, and plasma markers.

TREATMENT

Current treatment options can be categorized as the "3 Ds": drugs, diet, and dilation. These options can be used alone or in combination.

Diet

Given the proposed role of food antigens in disease pathogenesis, dietary modifications have been proposed for management. Dietary treatment strategies are implemented following initial endoscopy and biopsy. After following the proposed diet for a set time interval, systematic reintroduction of food allergens is performed gradually during the course of weeks to months. With this method, food allergen triggers are isolated and able to be avoided, allowing for induction and maintenance of disease remission. A histologic remission rate up to 65% has been reported by meta-analysis of retrospective and prospective dietary therapy studies in both adults and children.[30]

One such dietary therapy, the *elemental diet*, is a liquid diet of soluble basic nutrients, including amino acids, fat, sugar, vitamins, and minerals. Intact proteins are intentionally avoided, as proposed antigen triggers. Histologic remission in about 90% of patients has been reported with this method.[30] However, there has been less consistency in symptomatic improvement, particularly in adults.[31] Additional limitations of this diet include poor palatability, limited patient adherence, high cost, and social implications of liquid-only diet.

Elimination diet can be empiric, where most commonly associated allergic antigens are avoided during the treatment period. The *six-food elimination diet* (SFED) is the most popular of these, eliminating cow's milk, egg, soy, wheat, peanuts/tree nuts, and fish/shellfish. A meta-analysis of SFED demonstrated combined effectiveness of 72% with good homogeneity regardless of patient age.[30] Triggers were identified during the reintroduction phase using SFED in 30% to 35% of patients at the following frequencies: cow's milk, 61.9%; wheat, 28.6%; eggs, 26.2%; and legumes, 23.8%.[9] With continued trigger avoidance, remission was maintained up to 3 years.[9] Limitations of the diet center around lifestyle barriers and subsequent patient adherence.[32] Therefore, less-restrictive variations have been developed, such as *four-food elimination diet* and *two-food elimination diet*, with remission rates of 54% and 40%, respectively.[33,34]

Allergy testing-direct elimination diet is based on the thought that EOE is driven by allergic antigens through IgE-mediated and non-IgE–mediated mechanisms. Therefore, by conducting skin prick testing and/or atopy patch testing, food allergen triggers can be identified and eliminated. However, results show less benefit with this method. Overall, food allergy testing-based elimination diet induces histologic remission in less than one-third of adult patients. Additional studies assessing histologic response in adult patients with EOE show response rates of 22% to 36%.[30,35,36] Moreover, elimination diets have been shown to be equally effective in patients with negative skin prick results.[9,35] Therefore, the correlation between skin allergy testing and food allergen triggers is weak at best. Given this, studies have looked at the role of serum allergen-specific IgE in determining targeted diets. One study evaluating this found fewer foods needed to be eliminated, when compared to SFED, to achieve histologic remission but only when milk was the food trigger identified.[36] Other food allergen triggers resulted in similar response to empiric food elimination diet.[37,38] This means negative results on allergy testing neither rule out a specific trigger nor do positive tests pinpoint the effective dietary target, leaving currently a limited role for this dietary treatment modality.

Drugs

Proton pump inhibitor

Previously GERD and PPI-responsive eosinophilic esophagitis (PPI-REE) were thought to be distinct clinical entities, mutually exclusive of EOE. These were diagnosed by the presence of PPI response. However, more recently, GERD has been recognized as coexisting with EOE, and PPI-REE has been classified as a subtype of EOE. Therefore, PPI now acts as a first-line therapy option for EOE. This provides anti-inflammatory and acid-suppressive benefits. One meta-analysis identified histologic remission in 50% and clinical remission in 60% of patients on PPI therapy.[39]

This is the case even in patients without GERD symptoms and negative pH testing, although less common.[39] Current recommendation for the initiation of PPI therapy is omeprazole 20 or 40 mg twice daily for 8 to 12 weeks, followed by reassessment of symptoms and endoscopic visualization to determine the response. Long-term response to PPI is still unclear though. The first study assessing this, in 2015, showed loss of response on maintenance therapy in 27% of patients but most regained remission after dose escalation, and relapse in all 16 who temporarily discontinued PPI. Therefore, it is reasonable to implement a progressive taper of PPI dose to maintain remission.[40]

Topical steroid

Based on current guidelines, first-line therapy for EOE is topical corticosteroids. Remission has been demonstrated in adults and children with both fluticasone propionate and budesonide.[41] Significant reduction in histologic eosinophil counts has also been demonstrated.[42] However, this was only significant in patients not responsive to PPI. Therefore, topical steroids play less role in the management of patients with coexistent GERD. Additionally, there is less consistency in symptomatic benefit from use of topical steroids.[43,44] Comparisons of PPI (esomeprazole) to topical steroid (fluticasone) have found no significant differences in effect on dysphagia symptoms, degree of eosinophilic infiltrate, or histologic or clinical response.[45,46]

Topical steroid formulations vary but the most commonly used are fluticasone via metered-dose inhaler (440 mcg twice daily) and oral viscous budesonide (OVB, 1 mg swallowed twice daily). Drug to mucosal contact time is thought to influence treatment outcomes. This is supported by demonstration of histologic remission being higher in OVB versus nebulized budesonide groups.[43] Therefore, eating or drinking should be avoided for 30 minutes after medication administration. Then, a small amount of water should be gargled, swished in the mouth, and then spit out to rinse off any residue in the oropharynx and reduce the risk of oral thrush. A typical course of therapy is 8 to 12 weeks. Then, maintenance therapy is considered, particularly in cases with narrow-caliber esophagus, prior esophageal stricture requiring repeated dilations, severe or ongoing symptoms, or patient preference.[22] Topical therapy is generally considered low risk, without serious side effects. The main reported side effect is esophageal candidiasis.[47] Adrenal suppression has not been shown in an 8 to 12-week course of topical steroids.[48,49]

Systemic steroid

Systemic steroids have demonstrated increased histologic improvement when compared to topical steroids.[50] However, no clinical benefit has been demonstrated. Additionally, systemic steroids have a higher risk profile, with one study noting adverse effects (hyperphagia, weight gain, and cushingoid features) in 40% of patients, despite starting to taper at week 4 of therapy.[50] Therefore, systemic steroids should be reserved for short courses in refractory or severe cases.

Biologics

The role of biologics has been considered for EOE management. Given the role of IL-5 and IgE in disease pathogenesis, humanized monoclonal antibodies against IL-5 (reslizumab and mepolizumab) and IgE (omalizumab) have been proposed. Trials of reslizumab in pediatric populations showed a decrease in peak eosinophil count compared with placebo. However, histologic remission was neither achieved nor was there significant difference in endoscopic evaluation.[16] Trials of mepolizumab were unable to reach primary outcomes of histologic remission.[51,52] Omalizumab did not improve endoscopic or histologic features either.[53] Following these studies, additional biologics were further investigated. Currently, dupilumab, humanized monoclonal antibody against IL-4Ra, is Food and Drug Administration (FDA)-approved for EOE. Phase 3 trials demonstrated histologic improvement in about 60% of patients with weekly dosing, which was measured by the reduction of eosinophils to less than 15 per high-power field, as compared with placebo. Additionally, phase 3 trials demonstrated clinical benefit measured by improved scores on the Dysphagia Symptom Questionnaire in weekly dosing compared with placebo.[54]

Dilation

Esophageal dilation is a means to improve anatomic stricture or stenosis but it does not target the underlying cause of EOE. Despite this, a meta-analysis in 2017 demonstrated clinical improvement in 95% of patients undergoing dilation with minimum target diameter of 15 to 20 mm.[55] Symptom relief lasted for a median duration of 1 year. Complications included perforation (0.38%), hemorrhage (0.05%), and hospitalization (0.67%). No deaths were reported.

Consensus guidelines support performing conservative dilations as add-on therapy for ongoing symptoms. If critical strictures or food impaction exist, dilation can be used as a first-line therapy. Both through-the-scope balloon and bougie dilators can be used. With bougie dilators, tactile resistance and mild blood on the dilator can indicate sufficient dilation, which can be assessed with repeat endoscopy. Bougie dilators can also target longer segments of stenosis. The benefit of through-the-scope balloon dilation is the ability to visualize the mucosa during dilations without endoscope removal and reintroduction. Additionally, through-the-scope balloon dilation provides a static circumferential pattern of dilation, as opposed to shearing. Mucosal tear is expected and demonstrates the disruption of fibrotic remodeling, allowing for an increased luminal diameter. Esophageal luminal diameter of 15 to 18 mm is the goal. This should be achieved with less-aggressive, repeat interventions. Repeated dilations should be considered based on symptom profile.

SUMMARY

EOE is an immune-mediated disorder with increasing prevalence and significant burden. It is the leading cause of food impaction and dysphagia.[56] As of 2014, the annual health-care cost in the United States was estimated at US$1.4 billion.[56] Diagnosis depends on symptom history, endoscopy, and mucosal biopsy. Current treatment paradigms are efficacious in providing long-term benefit for patients, including dietary modifications, dilation, and medications. Emerging therapies continue to develop, such as the recent FDA approval of biologics. As the pathophysiology of the disease is better understood, more options will hopefully be developed in the management of EOE.

CLINICS CARE POINTS

- Prevalence in the United States is estimated to be from 30.9 to 71.9 per 100,000 cases
  - Highest prevalence in Midwest states
  - Male predominance
  - In adults and pediatric populations
- Pathophysiology involves IgE and non-IgE–mediated allergic responses, which drive a Th2 inflammatory response, resulting in release of IL-5 and eosinophil recruitment and deposition
  - Epithelial barrier impairment has also been implicated in EOE pathophysiology

- Symptoms include
  - Pediatrics: feeding intolerance, nausea and vomiting, and failure to thrive
  - Adults: dysphagia and food impaction, heartburn, and chest pain
- Diagnosis relies on acquiring adequate history, endoscopic findings, and multiple mucosal biopsies
  - Diagnostic biopsy contains esophageal eosinophilia of 15 eosinophils/high powered field ($\sim$60 eos/mm^2) or greater.
  - Biopsy alone is not diagnostic due to several other conditions that result in esophageal eosinophilia.
  - Treatment is based on 3 paradigms: diet, drugs, and dilation
  - Elemental diet is liquid diet of soluble basic nutrients, which is associated with high rates of remission. However, this is poorly tolerated by patients due to palatability, cost, and social implications.
  - Elimination diets aim to remove offending allergens and slowly reintroduce them in order to isolate triggers.
  - First-line medical therapy is topical corticosteroid (eg, fluticasone or budesonide). However, PPI should be considered in responsive patients or those with coexistent GERD.
  - Recent approval of dupilumab for EOE has allowed for targeted biologic therapy with promising results in clinical and histologic remission rates.
  - Dilation is reserved for symptomatic and anatomic management because it does not alter the underlying pathologic inflammation.

DISCLOSURE

The authors report no funding sources or conflicts of interest.

REFERENCES

1. Dellon ES, Jensen ET, Martin CF, et al. Prevalence of eosinophilic esophagitis in the United States. Clin Gastroenterol Hepatol 2014;12(4):589–96.e1.
2. Litosh VA, Rochman M, Rymer JK, et al. Calpain-14 and its association with eosinophilic esophagitis. J Allergy Clin Immunol 2017;139(6):1762–1771 e7.
3. Martin LJ, He H, Collins MH, et al. Eosinophilic esophagitis (EoE) genetic susceptibility is mediated by synergistic interactions between EoE-specific and general atopic disease loci. J Allergy Clin Immunol 2018;141(5):1690–8.
4. Blanchard C, Wang N, Stringer KF, et al. Eotaxin-3 and a uniquely conserved gene-expression profile in eosinophilic esophagitis. J Clin Invest 2006;116(2):536–47.
5. Lim EJ, Lu TX, Blanchard C, et al. Epigenetic regulation of the IL-13-induced human eotaxin-3 gene by CREB-binding protein-mediated histone 3 acetylation. J Biol Chem 2011;286(15):13193–204.
6. Alexander ES, Martin LJ, Collins MH, et al. Twin and family studies reveal strong environmental and weaker genetic cues explaining heritability of eosinophilic esophagitis. J Allergy Clin Immunol 2014;134(5):1084–1092 e1.
7. Attwood SE, Smyrk TC, Demeester TR, et al. Esophageal eosinophilia with dysphagia. A distinct clinicopathologic syndrome. Dig Dis Sci 1993;38(1):109–16.
8. Assa'ad AH, Putnam PE, Collins MH, et al. Pediatric patients with eosinophilic esophagitis: an 8-year follow-up. J Allergy Clin Immunol 2007;119(3):731–8.
9. Lucendo AJ, Arias Á, González-Cervera J, et al. Empiric 6-food elimination diet induced and maintained prolonged remission in patients with adult eosinophilic esophagitis: a prospective study on the food cause of the disease. J Allergy Clin Immunol 2013;131(3):797–804.

10. Swoger JM, Weiler CR, Arora AS. Eosinophilic esophagitis: is it all allergies? Mayo Clin Proc 2007;82:1541–9.

11. Spergel JM, Andrews T, Brown-Whitehorn TF, et al. Treatment of eosinophilic esophagitis with specific food elimination diet directed by a combination of skin prick and patch tests. Ann Allergy Asthma Immunol 2005;95:336–43.

12. Vicario M, Blanchard C, Stringer KF, et al. Local B cells and IgE production in the oesophageal mucosa in eosinophilic oesophagitis. Gut 2010;59(1):12–20.

13. Akei HS, Mishra A, Blanchard C, et al. Epicutaneous antigen exposure primes for experimental eosinophilic esophagitis in mice. Gastroenterology 2005;129: 985–94 [PubMed:16143136].

14. Cho JY, Doshi A, Rosenthal P, et al. Smad3-deficient mice have reduced esophageal fibrosis and angiogenesis in a model of egg-induced eosinophilic esophagitis. J Pediatr Gastroenterol Nutr 2014;59:10–6 [PubMed: 24590208].

15. Masterson JC, McNamee EN, Hosford L, et al. Local hypersensitivity reaction in transgenic mice with squamous epithelial IL-5 overexpression provides a novel model of eosinophilic oesophagitis. Gut 2014;63:43–53 [PubMed: 23161496].

16. Spergel JM, Rothenberg ME, Collins MH, et al. Reslizumab in children and adolescents with eosinophilic esophagitis: results of a double-blind, randomized, placebo-controlled trial. J Allergy Clin Immunol 2012;129(2):456, e1–463.e3. [PubMed: 22206777].

17. Rothenberg ME, Wen T, Greenberg A, et al. Intravenous anti-IL-13 mAb QAX576 for the treatment of eosinophilic esophagitis. J Allergy Clin Immunol 2015;135: 500–7 [PubMed:25226850].

18. Katzka DA, Tadi R, Smyrk TC, et al. Effects of topical steroids on tight junction proteins and spongiosis in esophageal epithelia of patients with eosinophilic esophagitis. Clin Gastroenterol Hepatol 2014;12(11):1824, e1–1829.e1. [PubMed: 24681080].

19. van Rhijn BD, Weijenborg PW, Verheij J, et al. Proton pump inhibitors partially restore mucosal integrity in patients with proton pump inhibitor-responsive esophageal eosinophilia but not eosinophilic esophagitis. Clin Gastroenterol Hepatol 2014;12(11):1815, e2–1823.e2. [PubMed: 24657840].

20. Sherrill JD, Kc K, Wu D, et al. Desmoglein-1 regulates esophageal epithelial barrier function and immune responses in eosinophilic esophagitis. Mucosal Immunol 2014;7:718–29 [PubMed: 24220297].

21. Remedios M, Campbell C, Jones DM, et al. Eosinophilic esophagitis in adults: clinical, endoscopic, histologic findings, and response to treatment with fluticasone propionate. Gastrointest Endosc 2006;63:3–12.

22. Dellon ES, Irani AM, Hill MR, et al. Development and field testing of a novel patient-reported outcome measure of dysphagia in patients with eosinophilic esophagitis. Aliment Pharmacol Ther 2013;38(6):634–42.

23. Schoepfer AM, Straumann A, Panczak R, et al. Development and validation of a symptom-based activity index for adults with eosinophilic esophagitis. Gastroenterology 2014;147(6):1255–1266 e21.

24. Safroneeva E, Straumann A, Coslovsky M, et al. Symptoms have modest accuracy in detecting endoscopic and histologic remission in adults with eosinophilic esophagitis. Gastroenterology 2016;150(3):581–590 e4.

25. Kavitt RT, Hirano I, Vaezi MF. Diagnosis and treatment of eosinophilic esophagitis in adults. Am J Med 2016;129(9):924–34.

26. Shah A, Kagalwalla AF, Gonsalves N, et al. Histopathologic variability in children with eosinophilic esophagitis. Am J Gastroenterol 2009;104(3):716–21.

27. Dellon ES, Liacouras CA, Molina-Infante J, et al. Updated International Consensus Diagnostic Criteria for Eosinophilic Esophagitis: Proceedings of the AGREE Conference. Gastroenterology 2018;155(4):1022–33.e10.
28. Spechler SJ, Genta RM, Souza RF. Thoughts on the complex relationship between gastroesophageal reflux disease and eosinophilic esophagitis. Am J Gastroenterol 2007;102(6):1301–6.
29. Liacouras CA, Furuta GT, Hirano I, et al. Eosinophilic esophagitis: updated consensus recommendations for children and adults. J Allergy Clin Immunol 2011;128:3–20.
30. Arias A, González-Cervera J, Tenias JM, et al. Efficacy of dietary interventions for inducing histologic remission in patients with eosinophilic esophagitis: a systematic review and meta-analysis. Gastroenterology 2014;146(7):1639–48.
31. Peterson KA, Byrne KR, Vinson LA, Ying J, Boynton KK, Fang JC, Gleich GJ, Adler DG, Clayton F. Elemental diet induces histologic response in adult eosinophilic esophagitis. Am J Gastroenterol 2013;108:759–66.
32. Wang R, Hirano I, Doerfler B, et al. Assessing adherence and barriers to long-term elimination diet therapy in adults with eosinophilic esophagitis. Dig Dis Sci 2018;63(7):1756–62.
33. Molina-Infante J, Arias A, Barrio J, et al. Four-food group elimination diet for adult eosinophilic esophagitis: a prospective multicenter study. J Allergy Clin Immunol 2014;134(5):1093–1099 e1.
34. Molina-Infante J, Arias Á, Alcedo J, et al. Step-up empiric elimination diet for pediatric and adult eosinophilic esophagitis: the 2-4-6 study. J Allergy Clin Immunol 2018;141(4):1365–72.
35. Molina-Infante J, Martin-Noguerol E, Alvarado-Arenas M, et al. Selective elimination diet based on skin testing has suboptimal efficacy for adult eosinophilic esophagitis. J Allergy Clin Immunol 2012;130(5):1200–2.
36. Wolf WA, Jerath MR, Sperry SLW, et al. Dietary elimination therapy is an effective option for adults with eosinophilic esophagitis. Clin Gastroenterol Hepatol 2014;12(8):1272–9.
37. Rodriguez-Sanchez J, Gómez Torrijos E, López Viedma B, et al. Efficacy of IgE-targeted vs empiric six-food elimination diets for adult eosinophilic oesophagitis. Allergy 2014;69(7):936–42.
38. Gonzalez-Cervera J, Angueira T, Rodriguez-Domínguez B, et al. Successful food elimination therapy in adult eosinophilic esophagitis: not all patients are the same. J Clin Gastroenterol 2012;46(10):855–8.
39. Lucendo AJ, Arias A, Molina-Infante J. Efficacy of proton pump inhibitor drugs for inducing clinical and histologic remission in patients with symptomatic esophageal eosinophilia: a systematic review and meta-analysis. Clin Gastroenterol Hepatol 2016;14(1):13–22, e1.
40. Molina-Infante J, Rodriguez-Sanchez J, Martinek J, et al. Long-term loss of response in proton pump inhibitor-responsive esophageal eosinophilia is uncommon and influenced by CYP2C19 genotype and rhinoconjunctivitis. Am J Gastroenterol 2015;110(11):1567–75.
41. Murali AR, Gupta A, Attar BM, et al. Topical steroids in eosinophilic esophagitis: systematic review and meta-analysis of placebo-controlled randomized clinical trials. J Gastroenterol Hepatol 2016;31(6):1111–9.
42. Chuang MY, Chinnaratha MA, Hancock DG, et al. Topical steroid therapy for the treatment of eosinophilic esophagitis (EoE): a systematic review and meta-analysis. Clin Transl Gastroenterol 2015;6:e82.

43. Dellon ES, Sheikh A, Speck O, et al. Viscous topical is more effective than nebulized steroid therapy for patients with eosinophilic esophagitis. Gastroenterology 2012;143:321–4.
44. Tan ND, Xiao YL, Chen MH. Steroids therapy for eosinophilic esophagitis: systematic review and meta-analysis. J Dig Dis 2015;16:431–42.
45. Peterson KA, Thomas KL, Hilden K, et al. Comparison of esomeprazole to aerosolized, swallowed fluticasone for eosinophilic esophagitis. Dig Dis Sci 2010; 55(5):1313–9.
46. Moawad FJ, Veerappan GR, Dias JA, et al. Randomized controlled trial comparing aerosolized swallowed fluticasone to esomeprazole for esophageal eosinophilia. Am J Gastroenterol 2013;108(3):366–72.
47. Schaefer ET, Fitzgerald JF, Molleston JP, et al. Comparison of oral prednisone and topical fluticasone in the treatment of eosinophilic esophagitis: a randomized trial in children. Clin Gastroenterol Hepatol 2008;6(2):165–73.
48. Dohil R, Newbury R, Fox L, et al. Oral viscous budesonide is effective in children with eosinophilic esophagitis in a randomized, placebo-controlled trial. Gastroenterology 2010;139(2):418–29.
49. Alexander JA, Jung KW, Arora AS, et al. Swallowed fluticasone improves histologic but not symptomatic response of adults with eosinophilic esophagitis. Clin Gastroenterol Hepatol 2012;10(7):742–749 e1.
50. Liacouras CA, Wenner WJ, Brown K, et al. Primary eosinophilic esophagitis in children: successful treatment with oral corticosteroids. J Pediatr Gastroenterol Nutr 1998;26(4):380–5.
51. Straumann A, Conus S, Grzonka P, et al. Anti-interleukin-5 antibody treatment (mepolizumab) in active eosinophilic oesophagitis: a randomised, placebo-controlled, double-blind trial. Gut 2010;59(1):21–30.
52. Assa'ad AH, Gupta SK, Collins MH, et al. An antibody against IL-5 reduces numbers of esophageal intraepithelial eosinophils in children with eosinophilic esophagitis. Gastroenterology 2011;141(5):1593–604.
53. Rocha R, Vitor AB, Trindade E, et al. Omalizumab in the treatment of eosinophilic esophagitis and food allergy. Eur J Pediatr 2011;170:1471–4.
54. Dellon ES, Rothenberg ME, Collins MH, et al. Dupilumab in Adults and Adolescents with Eosinophilic Esophagiti. N Engl J Med 2022;387:2317–30.
55. Moawad FJ, Molina-Infante J, Lucendo AJ, et al. Systematic review with meta-analysis: endoscopic dilation is highly effec- tive and safe in children and adults with eosinophilic oesophagitis. Aliment Pharmacol Ther 2017;46(2):96–105.
56. Jensen ET, Kappelman MD, Martin CF, et al. Health-care utilization, costs, and the burden of disease related to eosinophilic esophagitis in the United States. Am J Gastroenterol 2015;110(5):626–32.

Moving?

Make sure your subscription moves with you!

To notify us of your new address, find your **Clinics Account Number** (located on your mailing label above your name), and contact customer service at:

Email: journalscustomerservice-usa@elsevier.com

800-654-2452 (subscribers in the U.S. & Canada)
314-447-8871 (subscribers outside of the U.S. & Canada)

Fax number: 314-447-8029

Elsevier Health Sciences Division
Subscription Customer Service
3251 Riverport Lane
Maryland Heights, MO 63043

*To ensure uninterrupted delivery of your subscription, please notify us at least 4 weeks in advance of move.

Printed and bound by CPI Group (UK) Ltd, Croydon, CR0 4YY

03/10/2024

01040473-0018